INTRODUCTION

INTRODUCTION

CHAPTER 1: WHAT IS THE LEAKY GUT SYNDROME AND WHY YOU SHOULD CARE?

CHAPTER 2: GUT RELATED CHRONIC DISEASES

CHAPTER 3: GUT HEALTH AND MENTAL HEALTH

CHAPTER 4: HOW TO HEAL YOUR GUT?

CHAPTER 5: THE HEALTHY GUT DIET

CHAPTER 6: THE HEALTHY GUT LIFESTYLE ACTION PLAN

CONCLUSION

Resources Page

Breakfast Recipes

  Gut-Healing Smoothie

  Aloe-Mint Smoothie

  Cinnamon Berry Smoothie

  Spinach and Aloe Smoothie

  Berry Flax Smoothie

  Strawberry Healthy Gut Smoothie

  Apple-Banana Smoothie

  Turmeric Latte

  Herb Scrambled Egg with Asparagus

  Sausage and Sauerkraut

  Banana, Flax and Turmeric Oats

  Sweet Miso Porridge

  Buckwheat Pancakes

  Lemony Quinoa

Lunch Recipes

Beef and Veggie Burgers

Turmeric Cauliflower Soup

Chicken Pesto Pasta with Asparagus

Tomato-less Soup

Herb Bone Marrow

Smoked Salmon with Spinach and Lemon Salad

Baked Chicken

Grilled Sauerkraut Avocado Sandwich

Garlic Shrimp in Butter Sauce

Mushroom and Leek Soup

Chicken Meatballs with Greens

Veggie Stir Fry

Roasted Broccoli

Dinner Recipes

Veggies and Shrimp with Rice Noodles

Chicken Thighs with Pineapple Salsa

Salmon with Green Beans

Chicken Piccata

Creamy Potato and Chicken Soup

Superfood Burger

Taco Soup

Thai Chickpea Curry

Turkey Soup

Coconut Chicken Curry

Veggie Packed Soup

Beef Ragu with Spaghetti Squash

Almond-Crusted Cod with Greens

Desserts

Banana and Mint Chip Ice Cream

Baked Stuffed Apples

Poached Pears

Mango and Lime Sorbet

Salads

Sauerkraut Salad

Avocado and Papaya Salad

Mango and Red Cabbage Salad

Roasted Veggie Salad

Soups

Chicken and Chickpea Soup

Chicken Zoodle Pho

Mexicali Chicken Soup

Emerald City Soup

Butternut Squash Soup

INTRODUCTION

Current scientific evidence has suggested that a leaky gut triggers aplenty of medical conditions. The leaky gut syndrome or LGS is a digestive condition that damages the lining of the intestines. It is a condition where gaps in the walls of the intestine allow bacteria and other toxins to enter the body's bloodstream.

The gastrointestinal (GI) tract houses organs such as the esophagus, the stomach as well as the large and small intestines. This tract is a tube that runs from the mouth to the anus connecting several organs. The digestive process is carried out by this tract where digestive enzymes in our stomach and small intestines break down food nutrients into small pieces that are easily absorbed by the body for energy, growth, and repair of body tissues.

Our intestines help to protect the body from harmful bacteria and toxins. How the intestines do this? The tight openings in the intestinal walls give room for water and nutrients to pass through and go into our bloodstream while also keeping aside harmful substances. When someone suffers from LGS, these intestinal openings become wider, which gives passage to food particles, bacteria, and toxins to enter our bloodstream directly.

Our intestines house a range of bacteria called gut microbiota, which aid in the digestion process. They also protect the intestinal wall and gives support to the normal functions of our immune system. Suffering from Leaky gut syndrome may involve an imbalance of the gut microbiota. An article published in 2016 suggests that an imbalance in gut microbiota could trigger a response from the body's immune system. The effect is inflammation of the gut and an increased intestinal permeability, otherwise known as IP. Intestinal permeability helps describe how substances leak out of the intestine easily into our bloodstream. Research suggests that there is a link between leaky gut syndrome and other health conditions, including:

- Irritable bowel syndrome (IBS)
- Crohn's disease
- Celiac disease
- Chronic liver disease
- Diabetes
- Food allergies

- Food sensitivities

But it is still not clear whether LGS is a direct cause or a symptom of these conditions. However, in a review article published in 2015, the article suggests that an increased IP could develop into Inflammatory Bowel Disease or IBD. Also, another review article published in 2019 suggests that IP occurs before the occurrence of type 1 diabetes.

One of the possible causes of leaky gut, as suggested by medical practitioners, is an increased intestinal permeability. Sometimes, it is otherwise known as intestinal hyperpermeability. This condition occurs when the tight junctions in the gut responsible for the control of items that pass through the lining of the small intestine are no longer functioning like they ought to, the result of this scenario is that substances could leak into our bloodstream whether harmful or not.

It is most noticeable in people who have celiac disease or Crohn's disease. Either way, it is still unclear whether hyperpermeability serves as a more contributing factor to LGS or is merely a consequence of suffering from LGS. There is little knowledge about the causes of leaky gut that are not in one way or the other, linked to certain drugs, radiation therapy, or food allergies.

In more recent medical investigations, it has been discovered that scientists have also been investigating the relationship between the GI tract and our brains. A review published in 2017 suggests that leaky gut causes or contributes to the development of medical conditions like depression and anxiety. It has proven difficult for scientists to distinguish symptoms of the leaky gut syndrome because it shares many symptoms with several other health conditions.

Since the symptoms of leaky gut aren't unique, tests often fail to uncover the definite cause of the problem. Most often than not, people leave the doctor's office without a diagnosis and go on with untreated symptoms of leaky gut for a long time. Since doctors fail to get to the root of the problem when patients visit them, patients usually prefer to seek alternative medicine.

Some of the symptoms of suffering from leaky gut include:

A severe case of chronic diarrhea, constipation or bloating

- Nutritional deficiencies

- Fatigue
- Headaches and migraines
- Confusion
- Concentration difficulties
- Skin problems
- Joint pain
- Widespread inflammation

While these are some of the symptoms, it is still unclear what the causes and triggers of leaky gut are, but several risk factors can affect the gut microbiota and increase our IP. Some of these risk factors include:

- Poor nutrition
- Alcohol
- Body infections
- Autoimmune disorders
- Diabetes
- Stress

In many cases, leaky gut is triggered by what we eat. I used to eat unhealthy and packaged foods daily because of their convenience. Then after a lot of experimenting with changing my diet and long hours of research, I discovered that these kinds of foods were like strangers to my body, and my body decided that they needed to be fought off. My body then went to war and created antibodies to fight off these foods triggering an immune response that included fatigue, severe headaches, diarrhea, and pains in my joints.

Antibiotics, steroids, and over-the-counter pain relievers could trigger leaky gut. They irritate the linings of the intestine and damage the layers of protective mucus. This irritation could trigger or even continue the cycle of inflammation that leads to intestinal permeability.

Some experts claim that there is also a link between LGS and autism. While they are not sure how exactly autism develops, there are suggestions of the possibility that several genetic, biological, and environmental factors trigger this condition.

In 2016, a review stated that children who have autism develop digestive problems like constipation, diarrhea, and vomiting. Also, in 2019, research confirmed that there is a connection between gut microbiota imbalances and autism.

Since most medical practitioners do not think leaky gut is a legitimate medical condition but a rather fad diagnosis, there is no standard treatment for this condition. Diet is most likely a casualty of the leaky gut syndrome; hence, why you should see a gastroenterologist who is trained in nutrition if you notice symptoms of LGS occurring frequently.

There are, however, some dietary and lifestyle changes that help to improve gut health. These changes may also alleviate symptoms of leaky gut. Some of the nutritional tips that could help improve your gut health include:

Eating probiotics to improve beneficial gut bacteria

Eating vegetables and whole grains rich in probiotic fiber

Consumption of meat, dairy, and eggs less frequently

Stay away from added sugar contents and artificial sweeteners

Here are some lifestyle tips that can improve digestion as well as promote a healthy gut include:

- Regular exercise
- Sleeping well
- Avoiding stress
- Using antibiotics when necessary
- Quit smoking habit if any

Several treatment options have been recommended to victims of this condition by advocates of the leaky gut syndrome like diet books, herbal remedies, and other special diets. Still, you should be very careful of the kinds of treatment being offered to you by people claiming to be experts of the leaky gut syndrome.

Sometimes, treating underlying conditions such as Crohn's disease or celiac disease may help resolve the symptoms associated with the leaky gut syndrome. But most often than not, a doctor is unable to do anything to help a victim's condition without a firm diagnosis that there is evidence of the patient's condition of LGS. Chronic stress could be a risk factor of the LGS, too, which is why doctors advise that we should always attend to our stress either through the use of medications or meditation.

In summary, certain lifestyle improvements that help reduce stress as well as improve our diet are some of the best ways to improve the leaky gut symptoms, especially when your doctor has been unable to identify any underlying condition that serves as a trigger. So many chronic health problems are often as a result of an unhealthy lifestyle, and there are no pills to solve those problems.

You might have been struggling to get over this seriously devastating health issue, but nothing you've done to improve this condition has worked out the way you intended; it's okay. This book has been written to give you the necessary step by step information that will help you in the process of healing. I was able to control my leaky gut within a few months by adhering to new dietary and lifestyle changes.

If you have any of the symptoms mentioned earlier, I would advise that you get examined by your healthcare provider, so a treatment plan that fits your issues can be developed for you. A lot of research has been made to make this book a useful resource for you, so knock yourself out!

CHAPTER 1:

WHAT IS THE LEAKY GUT SYNDROME AND WHY YOU SHOULD CARE?

UNDERSTANDING GUT-BRAIN CONNECTION

The gut-brain connection or axis s the term used to refer to the network that connects the brain to the gut. These organs are connected both physically and biochemically in many different ways.

Neuron cells, which are usually found in the brain and nervous system, are responsible for telling our bodies how to behave. The human brain houses an approximate number of 100 billion neurons. It is quite interesting to know that our gut contains about 500 million neuron cells connected to the brain through the nerves in our nervous system. The nerve which helps to connect our gut to our brain is the vagus nerve. It sends signals in both directions, which suggest that the vagus nerve is an important organ in the gut-brain connection.

The gut and the brain are connected via chemicals, usually referred to as neurotransmitters. They are responsible for controlling our feelings and emotions. For instance, a neurotransmitter known as serotonin influences our feelings of happiness and helps to controls our body clocks. Most of these neurotransmitters are produced by the gut cells and several millions of microbes that live within our cells. The serotonin is mostly produced in the gut.

Our gut microbes also produce a transmitter known as gamma-aminobutyric acid (GABA). It is responsible for controlling our feelings of fear and anxiety. Experimental studies carried out on lab mice show that certain probiotics increase the production of GABA and reduce behaviors that are anxiety and depression-like.

The gut-brain connection connects through the immune system also, which is why the gut microbes affect inflammation. The gut and the gut microbes are important role players in our immune system and inflammation as they are in charge of controlling what enters the body and what the body excretes. Some certain bacteria in the body produce lip polysaccharide (LPS), an inflammatory toxin that causes inflammation if too much of it is passed from the gut and into the blood.

This occurs when the gut barrier begins to leak, allowing bacteria and LPS to enter into the blood. Having high LPS in the blood as well as inflammation are said to be triggers of many brain disorders, including cases of severe depression, dementia, and schizophrenia.

The gut-brain connection links anxiety to several stomach problems, and likewise, some of our stomach problems are linked to anxiety. The expressions "butterflies in my stomach," "nauseous," are used for a reason – they help express our emotions. The gastrointestinal tract (GI tract) is sensitive to our emotions, such as anger, anxiety, sadness, happiness, and every other emotion we feel. All of these emotions trigger symptoms in the gut one way or another.

Our brains have effects that are directly linked to our stomachs and intestines. When we think about food, stomach juices are being released in our stomach, even the food we eat gets into the stomach. Hence, we can conclude that our stomach or intestinal distress can be a casualty or trigger of anxiety, stress, or even depression because the brain and the gastrointestinal tract are connected intimately.

Sometimes, we often experience gastrointestinal upsets without being able to determine what the cause of the problem is. This is because of the gut-brain connection. For functional GI disorders, it could prove difficult to heal a distressed gut because one hasn't considered the role of our emotions and stress play in triggering gut distress. When we study how the gut and brain interact closely, we would easily understand why you feel nauseated even before you show any signs.

Psychological factors team up with physical factors to make us feel pain and other bowel symptoms. Psycho-social factors have a role to play in the physiology of the gut as well as gut symptoms. In essence, what I'm trying to say is that stress, depression, and other psychological factors affect the movement and contraction of the gastrointestinal tract, which worsens inflammation and makes one more susceptible to infections of different kinds. Research has concluded that people who suffer from functional gastrointestinal disorders feel more pain acutely than others because their brains respond more to pain signals discharged by the GI tract. Stress could worsen the pains.

If your stomach or intestinal problems such as heartburn, muscle cramps, loose stools are stress-related, then you have to watch out for the following symptoms and discuss them with your doctor. By doing this, you and your doctor will be able to device a means to which you can improve the symptoms as well as treatment options to help you deal with the stressors you are dealing with as well as treating your digestive problems.

Here are some of the physical symptoms you should look out for:

- tense muscles in the neck and shoulders
- headaches
- insomnia
- tremors
- shakiness
- loss of interest in sex
- weight-loss
- weight- gain
- feeling of restlessness

Some of the behavioral symptoms include:

- procrastination
- grinding the teeth
- difficulty in performing tasks

Change in the amount of food or alcohol consumed

Abnormal increase in the desire to be amongst people or to withdraw from people

- brooding
- rumination about stressful events

Some of the emotional symptoms include:

- crying excessively
- overwhelming pressure or tension
- relaxation problems
- feelings of nervousness
- mood swings
- quick temper
- depression
- concentration problems
- problem with remembering things
- loss of sense of humor
- indecisiveness

I would like to enlighten you on what you should know if you suspect you are suffering from the leaky gut syndrome or know someone who has this illness. Usually, the symptoms of the leaky gut syndrome are bloating, gas, cramps, food sensitivities, and as well as aches and pains, but the subject is still a medical mystery.

Many gastroenterologists are of the view that leaky gut syndrome is a gray area, as most physicians lack enough information about the gut, which happens to be the biggest organ in our immune system. This syndrome is not a diagnosis they teach in medical school, rather being a victim of this syndrome requires an even more accurate diagnosis before conclusions or speculations.

In the absence of evidence regarding the existence of this medical condition, there are no accurate therapies or prescription medications to address improvement in the symptoms that this mysterious syndrome happens to propagate. Dr. Donald Kirby, a gastroenterologist and director of the center for human nutrition at the Cleveland clinic says, "you hope that your doctor is good-enough Sherlock Holmes, but sometimes it is very hard to make a diagnosis."

Before the medical society understood the mechanisms that cause certain diseases, they believed that certain ailments were a result of imbalances in the stomach, referred to as hypochondriasis in ancient Greece. The upper part of the abdomen was referred to as the hypochondrium. Although, as science evolved, this notion was soon discredited. But this ancient belief that most illnesses originate from the gut may be worth some credibility. We can often conclude that some chronic diseases in today's society are a result of a dysfunctional gastrointestinal system.

The leaky gut syndrome is getting quite popular in medical blogs and even on social media in recent times. Still, it should not be so surprising if you discover that your doctor or physician is not aware of the term. The term leaky gut can also be referred to as increased intestinal permeability and is somewhat new in contemporary medicine as most research on the subject occurs in basic sciences. This, however, does not reduce the fact that leaky gut syndrome has developed growing interest globally, and medications are being developed for people with leaky gut to improve the effects of this condition.

What is the leaky gut syndrome all About?

In the belly of every human being, there is an extensive intestinal lining that covers about 4,000 square feet of surface area and more than forms a barrier that helps to control what is being absorbed into our bloodstream. Still, it is only able to perform this function when it is working properly. Having an unhealthy gut lining may cause the lining to have cracks and holes which allow food that has been partially digested to penetrate the tissues below the lining, including toxins and bugs.

The effect of this could trigger inflammation, including changes in the gut flora, otherwise known as normal bacteria. This could further lead to problems within and beyond our digestive tracts. Research gathered from across the world, showing modifications in intestinal bacteria and inflammation may affect the development of several diseases that are quite common.

You might be wondering: "who gets the leaky gut and why?"
To some extent, everyone has a degree of leaky gut, as this barrier cannot be said to be completely impenetrable. Sometimes, our genes have a

predisposition that may be more sensitive to changes in our digestive systems. In most cases, the contemporary lifestyle is to blame for gut inflammation.

there is convincing evidence that the standard American diet may trigger this process as it includes low fiber, sugar, and saturated fats, and let's not forget heavy consumption of alcohol by people who consume alcohol and stress. Stressors could trigger this imbalance of the body. We are all aware that increased intestinal permeability has a role to play in the development of some gastrointestinal conditions such as celiac disease, Crohn's disease, and irritable bowel syndrome (IBS).

But despite all these facts stated above, the big question on the minds of everyone is whether or not leaky gut triggers other health-related problem in our body system. Studies have shown that having a leaky gut could be a reason why people develop other autoimmune diseases like type 1 diabetes, chronic fatigue syndrome, arthritis, allergies, asthma, acne, obesity, or even mental illness. However, clinical studies were unable to show whether these happenings are that of cause and effect.

Physicians believe that people who have increased intestinal permeability are usually patients who have celiac disease or Crohn's disease. However, the conclusion is that increased intestinal permeability is a symptom of these ailments and not a cause, as some people believe.

intestinal permeability does not trigger anything beyond the general inflammation of the bowel walls and cannot be identified as the leaky gut syndrome. According to the advocates of the leaky gut syndrome, bacteria and toxins make their way into our bloodstream through the tight junctions and begin to damage the body system causing symptoms such as bloating, gas cramps, inflammatory bowel disease (IBD) including fatigue, food sensitivities, joint pains, mood swings, irritability, insomnia, autism and several skin problems like eczema and psoriasis.

But in truth, they are all speculations as scientific studies have continually failed to validate these claims. Many doctors who diagnose patients with leaky gut syndrome believe that a lack of adequate studies on the subject does not mean that the existence of this condition should be thwarted and debunked. Instead, they suggest that a more rigorous testing procedure be developed to support any new diagnosis as well as medications and treatment options before they recommend them to patients suffering from this condition.

How is it developed?

Our digestive tract is responsible for breaking down food and absorption of nutrients. Our digestive system also helps to protect our body from harmful substances hence, why the intestinal walls serve as barriers that control what does and does not enter our bloodstream as well as what is being transported to our body organs.

The small gaps in the intestinal walls, usually referred to as tiny junctions, give room for water and body nutrients to pass while also serving as a blockade against harmful substances. Intestinal permeability is how easily substances that have been absorbed move through the intestinal wall. When the tight junctions become loose, the gut becomes more permeable, allowing toxins and bacteria to pass through the gut and enter into the bloodstream. This phenomenon is called leaky gut.

When one suffers from leaky gut, these bacteria and toxins that should be shut out of the bloodstream make their way into the bloodstream and begin to trigger widespread inflammation and a possible reaction from the immune system. These responses are referred to as symptoms, and they usually include: bloating, food sensitivities, fatigue, digestive problems, and skin problems.

In sum, the leaky gut is a condition that is triggered when the tight junctions of the intestinal wall become so loose that toxins and bacteria make their way into the bloodstream of victims.

What are the symptoms?

When you suffer from the leaky gut syndrome, you are every likely to experience one or more of these symptoms:

- bloating
- gas
- cramps

- food sensitivities
- pin
- autoimmune disease
- thyroid problems
- inflammatory skin conditions or acne

What are the causes?

Like I mentioned earlier, the leaky gut syndrome is a medical mystery, and scientific research has still not concluded on the causes of the condition. The only fact that is known to help determine the cause of this ailment is a protein called zonulin, which regulates intestinal permeability. When this protein is activated in genetically susceptible people, it could cause leaky gut.

Some of the other causes of the leaky gut include

Poor diet

Unhealthy diets tend to create imbalances in the intestinal barrier, and some of these diets include

- low-fiber diets
- saturated fat diets
- western diets rich in fats and sugars
- processed foods especially those containing emulsifiers

Lectins

These are proteins that are concentrated in seeds such as grains, legumes, nuts, including tubers such as potatoes. Lectins prove beneficial since they stimulate the immune system, but they can sometimes bind to the surface of the gut-lining cells, which disturbs the gut barrier. Some dietary sources of lectin can open the tight junctions directly in the gut cells by increasing zonulin.

Injury

The more severe an injury is, the greater the increase in gut permeability. Studies carried out on 29 intensive care students showed an increased rate of intestinal permeability after 72 to 29 hours after suffering from trauma. Burn injuries are capable of causing leaky gut in both animals and humans. Studies show that rats and mice with traumatic brain injuries also had increased intestinal permeability.

Strenuous exercise

Exercise can increase intestinal permeability as blood goes into the muscles during exercise. The blood then moves away from the stomach, and the oxygen supply to the gut becomes reduced. Eventually, when the blood supply to the gut is reduced by more than half, there is an increase in intestinal permeability.

Alcohol

Consuming alcohol can affect the intestinal barrier function as well as increase gut permeability. Most alcoholics have higher gut permeability after four days of drinking and sometimes for two weeks. Consuming red wine moderately for one week is safe for healthy people but is capable of increased intestinal permeability in patients with active IBD. Some harmful bacteria produce alcohol, such as E.coli, which may be a reason why these bacteria compromise the gut barrier function.

Bacterial imbalance

This condition is also known as dysbiosis. Gut bacteria can alter the function of the intestinal barrier as a shield. When through gut microbiota is disturbed, the gut barriers suffer a dysfunction in several disorders and diseases.

Infections

When harmful bacteria like h. Pylori gain access to the body by altering tight junctions, they increase gut permeability. Other types of infection could trigger an increased intestinal permeability, as with the case of patients suffering from malaria. Patients suffering from malaria experience increased intestinal permeability.

Inflammation

People suffering from inflammation suffer n increased intestinal permeability through TNF-alpha, IL 1beta, IFN-gamma, Nf-KB, and other cytokines.

Drugs

Drugs such as the conventional NSAID increases gut permeability within 24 hours of ingestion. Some stomach acid-suppressing drugs are also factors that increase gut permeability. However, patients with cystic fibrosis, PPIs reduce gut permeability rather than increase them.

Zinc deficiency

Since zinc plays an interesting role in the maintenance of the intestinal barrier, a deficiency of zinc will increase gut permeability. Perturbed zinc balance is associated with abnormal gut permeability in children.

Deficiency in vitamins

Lacking vitamins such as vitamin d and a can trigger increased intestinal permeability. These vitamins are necessary for the intestinal barrier to function properly. Observational studies show that a vitamin a-deficient diet impaired the intestinal barrier in rats while mice deficient of vitamin d became more sensitive to gut barrier disruption.

Radiation

Being exposed to radiation such as radiation therapy increases intestinal permeability in human beings. In mice, being exposed to radiation disrupts the tight junctions as well as increase gut permeability. This also occurs in monkeys.

Chemotherapy

It is not fully understood "how" chemotherapy triggers an increase in intestinal permeability, but like radiation, chemotherapy increases intestinal permeability .

Infancy, formula, and breastfeeding

Babies are usually born with a leaky gut, which allows them to absorb immune substances present in the mother's milk. Pre-term babies have a more leaky gut than full-term babies two days after birth.

Babies that are being fed with formula tend to have a more leaky gut than babies who are breastfed.

Aging

As we age, our intestinal barrier tends to weaken. Gut permeability is higher in aging people. It is measured by zonulin. A study carried out on 215 adults showed that the gut barrier does not weaken with old age. Still, it deteriorates as a result of chronic inflammation and other minor diseases that become common as we age.

CHAPTER 2:

GUT RELATED CHRONIC DISEASES

When toxins can gain passage into our bloodstream, our bodies send signals to the immune system. These signals serve as a command to the immune system to protect the body from these toxins, and our immune system immediately takes to action upon receiving these signals. Each time our immune system responds to this signal, it triggers systemic inflammation. This is the reason why chronic inflammation is considered a primary symptom of leaky gut syndrome. When we suffer from inflammation, the body becomes unable to heal naturally, and it becomes easily exposed to several other diseases.

Research has shown that increased intestinal permeability can be associated with several chronic diseases. They include:

CELIAC DISEASE

It is sometimes called celiac sprue or gluten-sensitive enteropathy. Celiac disease is caused by extreme sensitivity to gluten. It is an immune reaction to gluten, which is usually found in wheat and cereal grains. Eating gluten triggers an immune response in the small intestine. If this continues frequently, this reaction from the immune system can damage the lining of the small intestine, causing malabsorption as the small intestine will be unable to absorb nutrients.

Some of the effects of malabsorption are diarrhea, fatigue, weight-loss, bloating, including anemia, and many other severe conditions. In children, this damage affects both the child's growth and development besides suffering from the observable symptoms in adults suffering from the same condition. However, children are more likely to experience symptoms not related to the digestive system as well as half the adults suffering from celiac disease.

Some of the symptoms include:

- Diarrhea
- Fatigue
- Weight loss
- Bloating and gas
- Pains in the abdomen
- Vomiting
- Nausea
- Constipation
- Anemia
- Dermatitis herpetiformis
- Mouth ulcer
- Headaches and fatigue
- Injuries in the nervous system
- Joint pains
- Hypersplenism

It has been discovered that people who have celiac disease suffer from increased intestinal permeability. The inability to absorb nutrients results in the following:

- Damage of the tooth enamel
- Weight loss
- Irritability
- Short stature
- Delayed puberty
- Neurological symptoms which include attention-deficit/hyperactivity disorder(ADHD)

Crohn's disease

Crohn's disease is an inflammatory bowel disease (IBD). This disease triggers a severe condition of chronic inflammation of the intestinal tract. The effects of this condition could cause abdominal weight, pain, severe diarrhea, fatigue, weightless, and sometimes malnutrition. When Crohn's disease triggers inflammation, different areas of the digestive tract can be affected.

It spreads deeps into layers that have been affected in the bowel tissue and can be debilitating and could also lead to even more severe complicated life-threatening diseases. There is no known cure to improve this condition, but there are some therapies that have been proven effective in improving symptoms as well as long-term improvements. Millions of people have been discovered to be doing fine health-wise with treatment.

Symptoms of Crohn's disease could be severe or mild, and development is usually gradual. Sometimes, the symptoms come without warning, and there are situations where no signs or symptoms are noticeable. Some of the symptoms of this condition include:

Diarrhea

Fever

Fatigue

Abdominal pain

Cramps

Bloody stool

Mouth sores

Loss of appetite

Weight loss

Pain near or around the anus

Inflammation of the skin as well as the eyes, joints, liver ducts and bile ducts

Delayed growth in children

Delayed sexual development in children

It is said that intestinal permeability plays an essential role in the development of this disease. Genetically, leaky gut plays a role in the development of Crohn's disease also. The cause of this disease is yet to be discovered, but doctors have continued to suspect diet and stress as the causes. Factors like heredity and a malfunctioning immune system could also be causes.

Diabetes

Type 1 diabetes is caused by the autoimmune destruction of pancreatic beta cells, which produce insulin. There is speculation that diabetes is triggered when toxins leak through the intestinal walls.

Irritable bowel syndrome

Also known as IBS, it triggers illnesses such as chronic diarrhea and chronic constipation. Increased intestinal permeability is a common illness in people suffering from diarrhea-predominant IBS.

Food allergies

Since suffering from leaky gut results in the passage of food proteins through the intestinal barrier, an immune response is triggered. This could be a form of food allergy. Also, food tolerances are associated with leaky gut syndrome by non-ige mechanisms.

Eczema

Large populations of Americans suffer from different stages and types of eczema. The term is usually used to refer to atopic dermatitis. It is the most common type of eczema in the world today. The word atopic means a collection of immune system-related diseases such as asthma and hay fever.

eczema symptoms vary depending on age, but it is mostly occurring in infants as dry and scaly skin patches.

Some of the symptoms noticeable in adults include:

Rashes in the elbow and knees and sometimes the nape of the neck

Permanent itchy rashes on the skin

Rash-related skin infections

In infants under the ages of 2 and children above age two till puberty experience slightly different symptoms, including:

Rashes on the scalp and cheeks

Extreme itches

Rashes behind the creases of the elbows and knees

Rashes on the neck, wrists, ankles, and the crease between the buttock and legs

Bumpy rashes

Light or dark rashes (rashes become thickened over time.)

There is no remedy for eczema, but there are several treatment options to heal the skin and prevent future symptoms. Treatment options are usually based on the age of the victim, including the symptoms and the victim's current health state.

While some people outgrow this condition, others don't. Eczema often causes the skin to suffer dry, flaky, and very painful patches, which can be very embarrassing and overwhelming. The main cause of eczema is an overactive immune system, and this is why doctors prescribe immunosuppressive drugs for patients, but this treatment option cannot be long-term since the consistent uses of immunosuppressant prevent the immune system from being healthy.

Recent studies have shown that the immune system can be rebalanced by restoring microbial balance, and the reason why this fact seems to be quite catchy is that people suffering from eczema have a decrease in microbial richness. It is still unknown whether restoring the gut microbe could be a relief to patients suffering from eczema.

Rosacea

Rosacea is a common skin condition that appears on the face. It is often mistaken for acne, eczema and sometimes, skin allergies. This infection is common among people that are fair in complexion and approximately affects about 14 million Americans. Although no cure has been developed yet, there are treatment options to improve this condition.

It results in the thickening and small pus-filled bumps on the face and is sometimes associated with a gastrointestinal condition known as small intestinal bacterial overgrowth or SIBO. Doctors have discovered that treating SIBO clears up rosacea.

People who have rosacea often discover that their symptoms disappear whenever they treat SIBO. This reversal in rosacea symptoms serves as an exciting development for those suffering from rosacea. It offers hope to victims looking to rid themselves of this infection.

Psoriasis

Gut dysbiosis often causes psoriasis. Psoriasis is a condition that causes the skin to experience painful scaly patches. Candida overgrowth, leaky gut syndrome, and inflammatory bowel disease are all triggers of psoriasis, and victims are more likely to have gut microbiome imbalances and higher levels of inflammation. Since dysbiosis and psoriasis are linked to inflammation, it has been suggested that therapeutic approaches for victims should involve re-establishing balance to the gut microbiome.

Dermatitis herpetiformis

Gluten intolerance usually causes this condition. It is often associated with changes to the lining of the small intestine like those of celiac disease, but it might not be the case that digestive symptoms are the cause of this condition.

This usually happens on the knees and elbows of victims of people with celiac disease. It appears in the form of a reoccurring rash and is usually caused by imbalances in the gut. The skin condition benefits from a change in diet, especially the removal of gluten from our diets.

Anxiety

Anxiety is another condition that is triggered by imbalances in the gut microbiome. But this condition can be improved by manipulating the gut microbiome. Studies have shown that an effective and powerful way to ease anxiety naturally is through the gut-brain connection.

Depression

Studies have shown that there is a connection between diet and gut health and mental health through the gut-brain axis. When there are alterations in the gut microbiome, one can begin to suffer depressive symptoms. It has even been discovered that some specific microbial species contribute to severe depression in people. This discovery has led to gut microbiome researches to be the latest and fastest-growing field in treating different psychological disorders. Doctors usually treat this condition with gluten-free diets and medication, and sometimes both.

Dementia and Alzheimer's disease

Alzheimer's disease is a disorder that wastes away brain cells progressively until it degenerates and dies completely. It is a common cause of dementia, a condition that results in a progressive decline in reasoning, behavioral, and social skills that affects a person's ability to perform independently.

Some of the early signs of Alzheimer's may include forgetfulness, especially forgetting recent events or discussions. As the condition continues to progress, such a person will develop memory impairment and then gradually lose the ability to perform the everyday tasks as he or she ought to. The medications that have been developed in place of Alzheimer's improve the symptoms temporarily or in most cases, slow the rate of declination.

These treatments can only help victims perform independently for a short period as well as the different programs and services that have been developed to help both patients and their caregivers. No particular treatment has been able to cure Alzheimer's or alter the declination process in the brain. As the case becomes more severe, complications such as dehydration, malnutrition ad infection could arise as a result of severe loss of brain function and even death eventually.

Several case reports have confirmed that the sixth leading cause of death in the U.S. is Alzheimer's disease. Several treatment options have been developed to treat this condition, but they have all been futile – no drug has been able to improve this condition successfully, and research has confirmed that the gut microbiome has a direct connection with the progression of this disease.

The gut microbiomes trigger metabolic pathways as well as inflammation, which also happens to be a casualty of dementia. Currently, several researchers are into the business of developing and exploring treatment options to treat Alzheimer's that begins in the gut.

Parkinson's disease

There is an undeniable link between the gut microbiome and Parkinson's disease. Emerging researches have continued to suggest that there is a connection between our gut health and Parkinson's disease. This discovery has led researchers to develop new therapeutic approaches to treat people with Parkinson's disease.

Autoimmune diseases

Autoimmune diseases develop when the immune system begins to attack healthy tissues. It has been confirmed that there is a direct link between dysbiosis and autoimmunity since 80% of our immune system inhabit the gastrointestinal tract. Dysbiosis leads to the breakdown of the gut's lining, and when the gut becomes leaky, unwanted particles begin to pass through unchecked.

The effect of this is inflammation, immune system dysregulation, and autoimmune diseases. It has been discovered via recent research that there is a rise in autoimmune diseases in the united states. These conditions are over 100, depending on the body tissues being attacked. Some of the most common autoimmune diseases are:

Graves' disease

Hashimoto's thyroiditis

Rheumatoid arthritis

Type 1 diabetes

Multiple sclerosis

Lupus erythematosus

Since leaky gut contributes to autoimmunity, a rapidly growing field of the autoimmune disease is influencing the gut microbiota.

Allergies

When your immune system begins to confuse certain foods or environmental factors as harmful pathogens, you have developed an allergy. The immune system reacts to these factors aggressively, and as a result, stereotypical symptoms such as having an itchy throat, runny nose, and red or watery nose are triggered.

Allergies are believed to be the result of gut microbiome diversity. Some of the factors that have been discovered to increase the prevalence of allergies are bottle feeding, cesarean factors, and blasting the gut microbiome with antibiotics.

Obesity

Obesity is a condition-based off of poor life choices and has currently reached epidemic proportions in the U.S. gut microbiome may make it nearly impossible for someone who is obese to lose weight. Dysbiosis has been discovered to exist in people that are obese, and the only promising possibility to improve this situation is to restore balance in the gut microbiome.

Type 2 diabetes

Type 2 diabetes is linked to gut microbiota very strongly. This is why recent therapies to improve this condition are focused on dietary changes. They are also targeted t the expressed genes of the gut microbiome and have been dubbed microbial genetics by advocates.

Osteoarthritis

It has been discovered to be the most common form of arthritis that affects millions of people globally. Osteoarthritis develops when the protective cartilage cushioning the ends of our bones begins to wear down. While osteoarthritis commonly damages the joints in the hands, knees, hips ad spine, osteoarthritis can damage any other joint in the body.

The symptoms can sometimes be managed, but the effects of the condition on the joints cannot be reversed. Constantly being active, weight-watching, and some other prescribed treatments could help slow the progression of the disease and even improve pain and joint function. Symptoms usually develop slowly; some of these symptoms include:

Pain

Stiffness

Tenderness

Loss of flexibility

Grating sensation

Bone spurs

Swelling etc.

Dysbiosis causes inflammation in the body, and osteoarthritis develops as a result of cartilage destruction and the inflammation of the joints. This effect eventually causes pain, and when the gut microbiome is balanced, there is n improvement in inflammation of the body. This is another reason why scientists continue to explore gut microbial balance as a means of preventing and treating osteoarthritis.

Colon cancer

Colon cancer usually develops from the large intestine, also known as the colon, the final part of the digestive tract. Colon cancer affects mostly the older adults and usually begins as a small, noncancerous clump of cells known as polyps. Polyps are formed in the colon. Over time, these polyps develop into colon cancer.

It is sometimes referred to as colorectal cancer, which combines colon cancer and rectal cancer. There are several treatments available to improve this condition, including surgery, radiation therapy, and drug treatments. Scientists have discovered that toxins that enter into the bloodstream produced two types of bacteria known as E.coli and B.fragilis, which combine in the colon damage the DNA of patients.

There are so many conditions associated with the gut microbiome, so it is advisable that pay more attention to what you feed your body with. If you feel like you are experiencing any of these symptoms, you should see your doctor and discuss dietary changes to aid the development of a treatment plan for your health.

CHAPTER 3:

GUT HEALTH AND MENTAL HEALTH

Earlier in chapter one, I mentioned a few things about the gut-brain connection. Many of us are not aware of our second brain. This second brain is hidden within the walls of our digestive systems and is located in our gut. This discovery has led to the revolution of the way medicine understands the connection between digestion, mood, health, and our thinking. This brain has been named the Enteric Nervous System (ENS). It is in two layers of approximately more than a hundred million nerve cells lining the gastrointestinal tract from the esophagus to the rectum.

What is gut-brain connection?

Many of us will be wondering what the gut-brain controls – it does not help you compose love letters if that's what you're thinking. But it does help control digestion. It is in charge of swallowing, the releasing of enzymes that break down food, the control of blood flow, which helps with the elimination and absorption of nutrients. The ENS doesn't control thoughts, but it communicates with our main brains to produce effective results.

In people suffering from Irritable Iowel Syndrome (IBS), the ENS could trigger emotional shifts as well as functional bowel problems like constipation, diarrhea, bloating, pain, and stomach upset. For many centuries, most physicians believed that anxiety and depression contributed to these problems, but recent research has shown that it is, in fact, the other way around. Contemporary studies have shown that irritation in the gastrointestinal system sends signals to the Central Nervous System (CNS), triggering mood changes.

These discoveries have helped explain why a higher percentage of people with IBS and functional bowel problems like constipation and diarrhea develop depression and anxiety. This newfound knowledge about the ENS-CNS connection better explains the roles of IBS and bowel-disorder treatment options such as antidepressants and mind-body therapies such as cognitive behavioral therapy (CBT) and medical hypnotherapy. Since both the big brain and our second brain are in constant communication with each other, therapies that work for either one will work for the other.

Sometimes, gastroenterologists prescribe certain antidepressants for IBS because they help calm the symptoms when these antidepressants act on the nerve cells in the gut and not because they feel that these symptoms are in the patient's head. Also, psychological interventions like Cognitive Behavioral Therapy (CBT) improve communication between our big brains and our second brain. Many healthcare experts have suggested that digestive system activity may affect our thinking as well as our memory – in other words, our entire cognitive activity, but it is only a theory as there is no concrete evidence to support this claim.

Another interesting topic is the discovery of how signals sent from the digestive system affect metabolism in humans. This is as a result of the communication between nerve signals, gut hormones, and gut microbiota, bacteria in the digestive system.

The gut and brain are connected through chemicals known as neurotransmitters responsible for controlling our feelings and emotions, especially serotonin. The microbes that live in our gut make other chemicals that affect the cognitive activity of the brain. The gut microbes produce lots of short-chain fatty acids like butyrate, propionate, and acetate. It produces these short-chain fatty acids by digesting fiber. These acids alter brain function in many different ways.

One of the ways includes reducing appetite. Studies have shown that consuming propionate reduces food intake and reduces brain activity also. Butyrate and butyrate-producing microbes also form barriers between the brain and the blood, which coined the term blood-brain barrier.

Gut microbes also metabolize both bile and amino acids to produces other brain-altering chemicals. The gut and its microbes control inflammation as the gut-brain axis is also connected via the immune system. The gut and gut microbes control what is passed into the body and what is excreted out of the body. If the immune system is active for too long, i could result in inflammation, which is known to be associated with a lot of brain disorders like depression and Alzheimer's disease.

Brain bacteria

In the field of neuropsychology and the study of mental health problems, there is a theory that bipolar disorder, schizophrenia, and many other psychological and neurological problems might be associated with alterations in the gut microbiome. These speculations have led to the conclusion that the disruption of the bacteria balance in the microbiome can cause an overreaction from our immune systems, which directly contributes to the inflammation of the Gastrointestinal (GI) tract. This further leads to the development of symptoms of disease that do not only occur throughout the body but also in our brains.

This connection between the GI tract and the brain is what is being referred to as a gut-brain connection or axis. There are speculations that infections that occur early in life have negative effects on the mucosal membrane in the GI tract, which affects the gut-brain axis and alters brain activity and development. This mucosal membrane can also be affected in other ways, including poor diet choices, radiation, chemotherapy, and the use of antibiotics.

The connection between anxiety and gut health

Psychological factors combine with physical factors to create pain and other bowel symptoms. In essence, stress, depression, and several other psychological factors affect the movement and contractions of the gastrointestinal tract (GI tract), including worsening inflammation and making us more vulnerable to infections. Further research in this area of interest suggested that some people suffering from functional Gastrointestinal (GI) disorders experience more pin than others who do not because their brains respond more to pain signals from the GI tract, and stress can worsen symptoms.

It is not wrong to expect that based on these observations, one would expect to treat functional GI disorders with therapies that reduce or remove stress, anxiety, or depression. It is, in fact, a working therapy, as several studies have shown that patients who received psychological treatment based on this approach experienced improvement in their digestive symptoms compared to those who received only conventional treatment.

Gut-brain connection, probiotics, and prebiotics

Since gut microbes affect brain health, changing gut bacteria is one of the reliable ways to improve brain health. Probiotics are live bacteria with so many benefits when it is consumed. However, probiotics vary.

Some probiotics affect our brain – they are usually called psych biotics, while some probiotics improve symptoms of stress, anxiety, and depression. Observational studies carried out on patients with irritable bowel syndrome and mild or moderate anxiety and depression that used a probiotic known as Bifidobacterium longum ncc3001 for a consecutive number of 6 weeks showed that their symptoms were significantly improved.

Prebiotics are mostly fibers that are fermented into the gut bacteria that also affect our brain's health. Several studies have shown that using a probiotic known as Galactooligosaccharides for three weeks reduces the number of stress hormones in our bodies, often referred to as cortisol.

The remedy

The key to restoring both gut and mental health is to maintain a strong balance that will favor beneficial bacteria in the digestive tract. First, you have to maintain a well-balanced diet that comprises food items that contain probiotic and probiotic ingredients. By doing this, these biotics will help to improve microbial health by restoring balance to the gut.

These are food items that contain live bacteria, and for prebiotics, substances that are rich in fiber should do the trick. Fiber should include those that nurture the growth of probiotic bacteria. You should watch out for readily available foods that supply different amounts of beneficial live bacteria grown during carefully controlled processes of fermentation. Some of these food items include common everyday items that we eat while others might be even more exotic but are readily available in supermarkets.

Probiotic food items include plain yogurt, kefir, cottage cheese, fresh sauerkraut, kimchi kombucha, apple cider vinegar, and miso. Also, one shouldn't cook, process, or preserve these probiotic food items at high temperatures as the probiotic effects of these foods could be lost and destroyed.

Probiotic foods do not contain living organisms, unlike its counterpart. Prebiotics foods improve the health of the microbiome because they contain indigestible fibers that ferment in the GI tract. These fibers are consumed by probiotic of live bacteria and converted to other substances that prove healthful to both gut and mental health. Prebiotic food items include artichokes, leeks, onions, asparagus, garlic, chicory, cabbage, asparagus, legumes, and oats.

Probiotic supplements are also helpful in the treatment of depressive symptoms as well as symptoms of depression, anxiety, obsessive-compulsive disorder, and other psychological and neurological conditions. Still, they must be used with the consent of a physician or a mental healthcare provider such as a psychologist or psychiatrist.

There are no standard recommendations for the use of probiotic supplements because researchers are yet to determine the kind of bacterial species or combination of species and doses that could help treat symptoms as well as ensure overall health. Scientists are not clear on whether single strains of probiotic bacteria are as effective as the mixture of different strains of probiotic bacteria.

Studies continue to look into the gut-brain axis, and the use of prebiotics to reduce symptoms ad occurrences of several mental health disorders as early research has proven positive, but a much larger population and human clinical studies are necessary to ensure the effectiveness of this treatment plan and how they can be best applied on patients.

CHAPTER 4:

HOW TO HEAL YOUR GUT?

Did you know that your body was designed to heal itself? The power that made our bodies can heal our bodies. If you've noticed, whenever you cut your finger, it bleeds then afterward; it forms a scab and then heals up completely. The body produces 2.5 million red blood cells every second and 250,000 white blood cells every second, and there are about 50 to 70 trillion cells in the human body, which is being controlled by the nervous system. The nervous system is the master control system of them all.

Are you also aware that one single neuron is responsible for as much as 833 impulses per second and that our liver performs over 657 functions at the same time? All these serve as evidence that our bodies can heal themselves. Our innate intelligence and incredible healing ability all started with two cells, one from each of our parents. It is, indeed, the biggest miracle! All processes, functions, and systems work harmoniously to keep our health in check. We have been specifically designed this way, which is why the body's healing ability is natural.

Stress

Now that we understand our healing ability, I'd rather consider it safe to say that the key to staying healthy is simple. As long as we keep obeying the laws of nature, the body will continue to heal itself naturally. However, the body cannot heal itself due to one particular element that keeps interfering with the body's healing ability. This element is stress, and this kills us more than we think.

Emotional stress: some of the causes of emotional stress are divorce, relationship stress, deaths, finances, occupational stress, unforgiveness, worry, anger, fear, depression, and indecisiveness.

Structural stress: causes of structural stress include acute injuries, all kinds of accidents, old wounds and injuries, burns, scars, arthritis degenerative, chronic pain, stiffness, excessive exercise, surgeries as well as the subluxations of other joints and the spinal cord

Biochemical stress: causes of biochemical stress include illness, infection, allergies, drug abuse, alcohol abuse, digestive disorders, inflammation, toxicity overload, and dehydration.

Energetic stressors: energetic stressors include poor sleep, insomnia, overwork, meridian energy imbalance, nerve interference, including emf stress.

All these stressors combine to damage the body's ability to heal itself. If we fail to put these stressors in check, our health will continue to deteriorate, causing us more pain, discomfort, and sometimes frustration. In sum, the effects of these stressors will continue to interfere with the ability to live our lives comfortably. However, there is a solution to this problem – one that has worked for thousands in the past. The solution is to uncover the causes of these symptoms and decrease the stressors through appropriate treatment options, which will then allow the body to continue healing itself naturally.

The moment we begin to restore balance in our structural, emotional, biochemical, and energetic systems, we will begin to experience good health. Some of the benefits of restoring balance include:

Pain relief

Improved energy

Improve vitality

Improved quality of life

Vibrant appearance

Ability to enjoy and participate in all kinds of activities and hobbies

The only way to enjoy the benefits mentioned above is by working on restoring balance in the body system. The process of restoration is quite easy and only requires that follow a simple process - a goal, a plan, a course of action and commitment.

Improving your gut health

Many factors could affect gut health. Some of these factors include diet, food intolerances, lifestyle, hormones, sleep, and medications. All these and many other contributing factors affect the state of how the body digests and excretes what you eat and drink.

In support of improving digestive health, I have compiled a list of highly recommended tips on how to heal your gut naturally. These tips have proven to be effective for thousands of victims. They include:

Use of probiotics

It is noteworthy to mention that there is a balance between good and bad bacteria within the digestive system. This balance controls the way our bowel functions and also aid in the elimination of toxins from the body. They also improve the body's ability to fight off infections and diseases as well as regulation of body metabolism.

It has been discovered that the gut microbiome plays a very crucial role in our overall wellbeing and health. Using both prebiotics and probiotics contribute to the improvement and balance of gut health. This is why it is recommended that one should consume both prebiotics and probiotics daily. Probiotics (good bacteria) are living microorganisms that reside in our gut. They support the body's immune system, including digestion, and aid the absorption of nutrients in the bloodstream. Probiotics are essential for maintaining gut health as they prevent the invasion of harmful microbes.

Use of prebiotics

Prebiotics help fuel probiotics as they are soluble fibers that feed good bacteria in the large intestine. They help in promoting good gut flora as well as healthy bowel function. When probiotics feed on prebiotic fibers, it produces a short chain of fatty acids which decrease the growth of disease-causing pathogens and help us maintain the health of the intestinal lining.

Natural prebiotics can be found in most plant-based foods; hence, we should be encouraged to eat whole food diets. Some of the rich sources of prebiotics are leafy greens, citrus, leeks, flaxseed, apples, and other organic foods.

Ginger tea

Drinking ginger tea has many benefits to offer the body and has been used for more than two decades to treat digestive issues. Ginger helps to relax the smooth muscles of the intestine, which helps to relieve symptoms of gas and cramping. By speeding up the movement of food into the small intestine, ginger also aids in stimulating proper digestion. Ginger is also very useful in eliminating any eating discomforts and can stimulate the saliva, bile, and gastric enzymes that aid in the digestion of food.

Aromatics ad anti-inflammatory cooking ingredients

Vegetables like carrot, which contain vitamins a, b complex, c, d, e, k, fiber, potassium, and many other nutrients useful to the body, support healthy digestion, including healthy metabolism, constipation, and stomach ulcers. They also reduce inflammation and improve skin health as well as good vision.

Cabbage juice can also help to maintain the strength of the intestinal lining and improves digestive symptoms like bloating and constipation. Garlic is also useful because it is antimicrobial and antifungal. Hence, ginger detoxifies the body and helps to maintain gut flora balance, including boosting immune function.

Eat more whole foods

Diets that are plant-based ad are rich in anti-inflammatory sources help improve gut health. These diets should include lots of fresh vegetables, salads, fish, and a healthy quantity of heart-healthy fats produced from olives and oils.

One of the essential elements of good health is a good diet. It gas played a very important role in supporting good health. This is why we have to consider what we eat or drink and how they affect our body either positively or negatively.

Treat infections

Another way to improve gut health is by treating any infections and dealing with the overgrowth of bugs. Parasites and small bowel bacteria alter the proper functioning of the gut. These kinds of infections must be treated properly if you truly want to heal your gut and live healthier.

Get rid of food allergies

If you notice that your body is sensitive to some kinds of food, you have to eliminate them from your diet. Foods like gluten, dairy, yeast, corn, soy, eggs should be monitored, and you should pay attention to how your body reacts to this kind of food as well as how you feel in the gut and what happens to other symptoms that you experience.

Exercise

It is true that exercise is good for your health but are you also aware that exercise can make you feel good also? Getting the right amount of exercise helps rev up your energy levels and even improve your mood. One of how exercise helps in improving gut health is by modifying inflammation. When there is inflammation in the gut, such a person is liable to suffer from either Irritable Bowel Syndrome (IBS) or irritable bowel diseases.

Exercise might seem inflammatory when it is done on a short-term basis but is a very powerful anti-inflammatory agent in the long run. Note that exercise will only work if you don't make it another stressor in your life. Studies have shown that regulated exercise cause contractions in our muscles, which will then release anti-inflammatory myokines, which are effective in fighting off pro-inflammatory signals from the fat tissues in the patients of bowel disorders.

Yoga is one exercise that comes with benefits for gut problems since yoga has to do with mind-body practice. Research has shown that a large number of gut disorders have a mental element and so yoga appears to be beneficial as long as participants keep up with their yoga practice. In sum, research has proved that exercises that are gentle and non-stressful are therapeutic enough to improve even the most severe cases of gut diseases.

CHAPTER 5:

THE HEALTHY GUT DIET

WHAT IS DIET?

Here's a quick question – what comes to your mind first when you hear the word diet? I'm sure you think diet means to cut short some food items or to lose weight. Most people are quick to suggest that the word diet has something to do with weight-loss or things not to eat, but they are wrong. Oftentimes, people misunderstand and misuse the word, which is why I have decided that in this chapter, i will give what the true meaning of diet is and why you need to approach this term from a different angle and perspective.

You must have heard about the long list of weight-loss diets. Many of us must have attempted to practice some of these diets. They include crash diets, low carb diets like the Atkins and dukan low-carb diets, low-fat diets, low-calorie diets, very low-calorie diets, fit for life diets, weight watchers diet, etc.

Many of us feel the need to go on a diet or to be part of the latest diet trend, and sometimes, you might wonder if it is time to change to a new diet. Well, the most important thing is that we eat something and when you eat, you have a diet. It's as simple as that! We are all on a diet.

To cut a long story short, the word diet means to eat. I'm sure you know that the moment we stop eating, we are less than a lifetime close to death. This means that if we do not diet, we will die. Hence, any food you eat is your diet. Diets should be associated with anything that involves our normal or recommended way of eating for healthy living and does not require us to resort to such extremes as the diet plans mentioned earlier. It is high time we viewed the word diet with a healthier approach. Everybody goes on a diet from time to time, but the problem is that we also go off diet too.

Here are some of the misconceptions of diet i would like to clear up:

Diet refers to your overall eating habits rather than dieting.

Dieting refers to something you do and tries for a specific period – it could be for a week, a month, or until you lose weight. Everyone can have a diet, but we do not necessarily need to diet. It is best to improve your actual diet and incorporate healthy changes to your lifestyle so that these changes eventually become a part of your normal lifestyle. Having a dieting mentality will not help with the last weight-loss and improvements with your health.

When you starve yourself, you slow down your metabolism. Instead, you should eat foods with fat and protein that will satisfy you. Learning to listen to your body is an invaluable tool in improving your weight and your health.

You can eat as much fruits as you want.

It is healthy to include fruits in our diet along with the whole and real foods, but when you're attempting to reduce your weight, you should also consider the level of your fruit intake. The reason is that fruits contain sugar, which is quickly digested by the body. Without a doubt, fruits contain nutrients as well as fibers, which are good for our health, but it doesn't mean you should begin to see fruits as free food. You should consider the number of fruits you consume when attempting weight-loss – sticking to one or two serving fruits and paying attention to your veggies.

All calories are the same.

No! Not all calories are the same. It is quite okay to not want to over-consume calories, but you don't need to count them since they are not equal. So many things influence the number of calories we consume and how our body processes them, including our hormones, emotions, cravings, and even our social schedule. Diets that make you restrict calories cannot be maintained as your body needs calories to function. This way, you are resting your metabolic rate. Your body needs a certain amount of calories to keep you alive.

Low-fat foods are the best alternatives.

If you remove all fat from your diet, including heathy fats, you are left with something that lacks flavor. This is why products that promise reduced fat should always include that they've added more sugar. A moderate healthy fat goes a long way and can help us burn fat.

The key to weight-loss is a glutton-free diet.

Being glutton-free increases weight loss, agreed, but when was the also time anyone you know told you that their glutton-free lifestyle has helped them drop their weight? You don't necessarily have to be glutton-free unless you have a medical reason to do so to reap the benefits of weight-loss. Healthy diets comprise vegetables, fruits, lean proteins, healthy fats, and some grains that are low in glutton. It is much healthier to stick to naturally glutton-free foods rather than feeding on processed foods that contain additives.

Also, many people pay too much attention to the number they see on the scale every morning.

If you focus more on working out instead and eating healthy, you might be gaining weight, but you will be developing a healthier body. Pay more attention to your eating habits consistently to ensure that you are eating healthy and use a pair of jeans or a little dress to measure your weight.

Are carbs bad.

no! Carbs are not bad for your body. The only thing you should worry about is the amount you consume – just like anything else, too much of carbohydrates will cause weight gain. Carbohydrates supply the body with four calories per gram. There are different types of carbohydrates, simple and complex; both are necessary for a healthy diet.

Fluids and beverages do not affect your health and do not cause you to gain weight.

If you are consuming a lot of sodas or other types of liquids that are adding calories to your daily diet, you have to reduce your intake or abstain from them completely. Sodas and high-calorie drinks such as coffees with additives add hundreds of empty calories to your daily intake and do not give your body the necessary nutrients. You should drink half your weight in ounces and enough water, but if you are unable to consume a lot of water, it is okay to drink any kind of non-caloric fluids.

Good nutrition takes time, so you will have to take baby steps every day to incorporate healthy changes into your eating habits. Eventually, these small steps will yield huge results. Some extreme diets may suggest otherwise, but everyone needs a balanced diet comprising protein, fat, carbohydrates, fiber, vitamins, and minerals in our diet to maintain a healthy body.

The need for moderation

There is no need for you to eliminate any category of food from your diet; instead, you should select the healthiest options from each food category. At the end of every meal, you should feel satisfied and not stuffed. Some people believe that being moderate means eating less, but that doesn't have to be the case.

banning some certain foods might cause you to crave them even more, and then when you can't keep up with the ban, you begin to feel like you have failed. Rather than placing bans, reduce the portion of unhealthy foods, and try not to eat them as often. The moment you being to reduce the intake of these foods, you begin to crave the less and start to think of them as occasional indulgences.

When eating, eat small portions of food. Visual cues can help with portion sizes when serving. By serving food into small plates or bowls, you can even trick your brain into thinking you=re eating a large portion of food. If you don't feel satisfied after eating, add more leafy greens or even top the meal with fruits. Also, learn to eat slowly and stop eating before you begin to feel full.

Being moderate doesn't mean that you shouldn't eat the kinds of food you love, but they should be consumed less, especially unhealthy food items. You only need to eat as much as your body requires of you and nothing more.

Overhauling your diet at once might be a recipe for disaster rather than doing that, why not try to incorporate some of the healthy eating tips mentioned throughout this book in your lifestyle from time to time till it becomes a part of your eating habit. Moderate healthy eating makes a significant impact on making your overall diet healthier and more sustainable without a drastic change in your habits.

So, what should you eat?

The walls of the intestine consist of tiny cells known as the epithelial cells. The gaps in between epithelial cells give room for water, ions, and many other nutrients to flow from the intestines into the bloodstream. Normally, food particles and wastes are not allowed to pass through these gaps, but as the case is with leaky gut, these gaps are expanded as a result of inflammation and bacterial imbalances in the gut.

When this happens, harmful substances gain passage into the body via our bloodstream. Research has shown the people who have low biodiversity of gut bacteria tend to experience inflammation. The effects often trigger other harmful conditions such as inflammatory bowel disease and obesity. This is why a diet that helps increase gut bacteria diversity will benefit the patients of the leaky gut syndrome.

Since the leaky gut is not an official medical diagnosis, there is no recommended treatment option for patients. Do not worry; there is a lot of ways people with leaky gut syndrome can help themselves and improve their condition as well as their digestive health. One of these ways is to maintain a diet that aids the growth of beneficial gut bacteria.

Most of these diets incorporate mostly prebiotic and probiotic foods that support the growth and development of beneficial gut bacteria. Some of these foods include:

Probiotic yogurt

Roots and tubers such as potatoes, sweet potatoes, yam, squash and turnips

Kefir or fermented yogurt

Fermented foods like kimchi, sauerkraut, and miso

Sourdough bread

Some cheeses

Vegetables like the eggplants, broccoli, cabbage, carrots, zucchini

Fruits like the likes of blueberries, grapes, oranges, papaya, strawberries, mandarin, lemon, lime, passion fruit, pineapple, coconut, oranges, and bananas

Nuts and seeds like almonds, peanuts, cashews, and pine nuts

Dairy products that are lactose-free and dairy-based like hard cheese, lactose-free milk, and plant-based milk products

Sprouted seeds like chia seeds, flax seeds, sunflower seeds and so on

Gluten-free grains such as buckwheat, amaranth, brown rice white rice, sorghum, teff, and gluten-free oats

Avocados, avocado oil, coconut oil, extra virgin oil and healthy fast are good for this condition

Meat and eggs are not left out either. Lean cuts of chicken, lamb, beef, turkeys including eggs should do the trick

Herbs and spices

Cultured dairy products like kefir, yogurt, traditional buttermilk, and greek yogurt are also helpful dietary options

Grains like oats, corn, rice, and guinea are good options too

In sum, diets that improve our digestive health should consist mostly of fibrous vegetables, including fruits, fermented vegetables, cultured dairy products, healthy fats, and finally, lean and unprocessed meals.

What are the foods to avoid?

Patients with painful gastrointestinal symptoms should avoid foods that are quite difficult to avoid. Most experts refer to these kinds of food as fermentable oligo-, di-, monosaccharides, and polyols are otherwise known as fodmap s. They are a short chain of carbohydrates that are broken down or fermented by bacteria. The result is the production of gas, which triggers bloating and flatulence. Some of these fodmaps are:

- Fructose
- Lactose
- Fructans
- Polyols

Experts have suggested that consuming low fodmap diets help to reduce the production of gas. These will then ultimately arid patients off the digestive symptoms that are triggered by the effects of the leaky gut syndrome. Some of the high fodmap diets that one should avoid are:

- Apples, cherries, peaches, pears, dates, goji berries and watermelons

- Some vegetables like asparagus, mushrooms, onions, and garlic
- Legumes like black beans, fava kidneys, kidney beans and chickpeas
- Both natural and artificial sweeteners like the likes of fructose, honey, sorbitol and xylitol
- Grains like wheat, flour, barley, rye and almond meal
- Some beverages like soda, fruit juice, beer, and wine are harmful too
- Other foods that may harm the gut bacteria as well as triggering symptoms of the leaky gut like bloating, constipation, and diarrhea are:
- Wheat-based products such as bread, wheat flour, couscous, etc.
- Junk foods like potato chips, candy bars, sugary cereals, etc.
- Snack foods such as crackers, popcorn, pretzels, muesli bars.
- beverages include soda, fruit juice, beer, and wine.
- Dairy products like milk, cheese, ice cream, etc.
- Processed meats like bacon and hot dogs or even deli meats and cold cuts.
- Refined oils like sunflower, soybean oils, including safflower oils.
- Artificial sweeteners like aspartame, sucralose, and saccharin
- Sauces like hoisin sauce, teriyaki, soy, and even salad dressings
- Baked goods like our everyday cakes, muffins, and pizzas may harm our gut bacteria.

Avoiding these kinds of food helps to reduce digestive symptoms as well as improve our gut health.

How to help yourself?

It is possible that in some people, certain foods are more likely to trigger symptoms more than other kinds of food. It could be helpful to use a food journal to keep track of one's dietary habits as well as the symptoms they experience and to point out the trigger foods that trigger their symptoms.

Here's a helpful meal plan for you:

For breakfast, you can choose to have either a fruit parfait of Greek yogurt mixed with blueberries, strawberries, and slices of kiwifruit or oatmeal of dairy-free milk or water with rolled oats topped with blueberries or just have a simple breakfast of eggs and toast. You can have some sourdough toast with one or two eggs to start your day.

For lunch, you can have a salad comprising mixed greens, sliced chicken breasts with carrots, tomatoes, or shredded parmesan cheese to top it off. You could also have frittatas made of eggs, broccoli, tomatoes, and any kind of protein – it depends on you! Of course, stir fry isn't off the menu either. You can choose to mix beef, broccoli, carrots, bell peppers, and zucchini noodles for your stir-fry lunch.

Other options for lunch are lemon chicken made of grilled chicken breasts with sweet potatoes and brussels sprouts or have a salmon either grilled or pan-seared with a side salad to top it off. If you must-have snacks, there are some healthy options for you.

Rice crackers with peanut butter, grapes, and brie

A combination of almonds, walnuts, and hazelnuts will serve as good snack options.

CHAPTER 6:

THE HEALTHY GUT LIFESTYLE ACTION PLAN

MINDSET AND WHY IT MATTERS TO YOUR HEALTH

Did you know that your beliefs have a significant impact on your success or failure regardless of the field or matter?

Our mindset shapes the life we lead, our actions, and the future possibilities of our world and existence. According to psychologists, our beliefs have an essential role to play in what we want or desire to achieve. The conclusion after several types of research has suggested that it is mostly our mindset that determines whether we will succeed or fail. But you must be wondering – what is a mindset?

Mindset asks whether we believe that qualities such as intelligence and talent are fixed or can be changed. People either have a fixed mindset or a growth mindset. People who have a fixed mindset believe that these qualities are inborn, fixed and cannot be changed, but those with a growth mindset think that the

Se qualities can be developed and improved through commitment and hard work.

Mindset can be described using eight principles. They are:

Mindset as a habit of mind

The word mindset was first used in the 1930s to refer to habits of mind that have been formed by previous experiences. In other words, mindset refers to deep beliefs, attitudes, and assumptions about ourselves and our perception of the world.

Experiences shape mindset

Our experiences create our mindsets. The distinctions we make about our experiences help us build our mindset. From every experience we encounter, we make different distinctions and develop different mindsets.

Mindsets expose us to blind spots

Allow us to view the world in fragments and never with the complete facts of existence. Every individual sees the world through the filter of their mindsets, and no one ever has a perfect mindset.

Mindsets are self-deceptive

An individual will encounter powerful opposition the moment they decide to shift their mindsets. Some of these oppositions are the tenancy for one to experience confirmation bias. This involves searching for and recalling information that helps reconfirm previous or pre-existing beliefs.

Mindsets help shape our daily lives

As we make our mindsets, our mindsets are also responsible for making us too. Our mindsets develop each of our thoughts, words, actions, and our entire lifestyle. If we ever decide to change our pattern of living or our lives entirely or just become more creative and improve our total wellbeing, we must have shifted from our pre-existing mindset.

Mindset helps in creating the world we share

Mindset is a powerful force for cultural and systemic change. If we want to create the world we live in more consciously, we have to be prepared to shift our mindset

Mindsets evolve from simple to complex

Mindsets can be developed in complexity as the more developed our mindsets become, the more we submerge into deeper levels of wisdom, including effectiveness in the world. Every individual's mindset evolves from simple to complex, static to dynamic, and from ego-centric to socio-centric and finally, world-centric. This evolution improves our ability to take perspectives, our ability to embrace ambiguity, and hold paradox.

Mindsets can transcend

Utilizing the power of mindfulness, every individual can transcend their blind spots and self-deceptive forces. They can also examine how their habits of the mind unfold to create their lives, including the world around them as well as tapping collective capacity for profound personal and social transformation.

In essence, we cannot avoid the far-reaching effects of mindset. It

Has a hidden web of influence that permeates everything all the time, including our beliefs, attitudes, assumptions, which manifest on the outside to shape the future possibilities on us and the world around us.

Mindset matters

That we've understood the principles that describe our mindset, we can now move on to why mindsets matter a lot. So here's the question you should ask next – why does mindset matter?

Beginning to examine our mindsets can trigger subtle but radical clicks in our minds when all of a sudden, we begin to

Experience new ways of seeing, being and acting. These shifts in mindset transform our lives meaningfully in many surprising yet fulfilling ways. The habit of developing a mindset is especially useful when trying to heal physical illness.

People may not find this enough reason to dig deeper into the nature of their mindsets, but the

Re is an even deeper and convincing reason to examine the habits of our minds. It is especially true that we are living in a turbulent time, and every person is dealing with different challenges – even ones they've never encountered before. The world is faced with increasing numbers of both social and ecological crises that worsen and intensify progressively.

We are not aware that our mindset is the ultimate cause of the many challenges and

Problems we battle either individually or collectively. All of the global challenges the world encounters today are a consequence of continually reliving the unexamined habits of the mind.

Three basic types of mindset

Everyone has a unique mindset, but there are some common mindsets that we have to be consciously aware of, and there are three of such mindsets. They are the fixed, growth, and benefit mindsets, which reflect our

Common beliefs about the nature of learning and leadership.

Fixed mindset

Fix minded people believe that their basic intelligence and talents are fixed traits and are therefore unchangeable. It is symbolized by the everyday expert whose goal is to look as smart as possible at all times and never appear dumb. They only believe they have a certain amount, and that is that for them – they don't intend to go further.

Growth mindset

People with a growth mindset believe that their abilities and intelligence can be improved and developed through conscious effort, hard work, and persistence. They do not believe that everyone is the same or that everyone can be a genius like Einstein, but they share the opinion that one's intelligence can be worked on and improved. An example of a growth mindset is people who continue to learn and develop themselves long after they finish their formal education.

Benefit mindset

Those who have developed a benefit mindset do not only want to fulfill their potentials but also fulfill them in such a way that society will benefit from his achievement? They question their actions and believe in doing good things for good reasons also. The benefit mindset can be symbolized by the everyday leader.

Let's assume that I have a difficult problem to solve and that

the problem is a challenge for me or a possible learning experience. Others may feel that the problem is impossible to solve. You will observe that i am operating a growth mindset. I believed i could learn and develop the skills to solve the problem.

Having a growth mindset

Is the key to success because, with a growth mindset, you believe that you are in control of your ability and that you can learn and improve your abilities. Having a fixed mindset simply means that your brain becomes active when you are being given a piece of information about how well you have done. In contrast, when you have a growth mindset, your brain becomes active when you are being told what you can do to improve their situation. The fixed mindset is about how they are perceived while the growth mindset is usually about how they can learn.

Our brains can change. In other words, you can change your mindset. The term for this effect is called neuroplasticity. Our brains are developed like plastic, which is why we can easily reshape our brains over time to form neural pathways. This is why neuroscientists regard this tendency of the brain to change as neuroplasticity. When the brains are subjected to change, the neural pathways begin to develop as we continue to engage in various activities.

our mindsets are not just for learning new skills; they also affect the way we think and deal with different situations. Our mindset is crucial in how we cope with our different life challenges

, including our abilities to heal from chronic illness such as leaky gut syndrome. When we are faced with problems or diseases, developing a growth mindset will help us show greater resilience and help us to persevere in times when we encounter setbacks. On the other hand, those who have developed a fixed mindset over time will be prone to giving up on their health very easily, and therefore they cannot overcome the illness.

How to build healthy habits?

You might have heard that conventionally, it takes one about four weeks to develop and maintain a habit. But I often wonder if that speculation is true or false. So that begs the question, how long will it take one to maintain and develop a healthy habit if you're trying to eat more nutritiously or live an anti-aging lifestyle?

No doubt, establishing regular healthy habits and breaking bad ones improve the longevity of life. The moment you begin to quit unhealthy behaviors like smoking drinking and practice healthy habits regularly, you will discover that it becomes easy to maintain these habits as well as entrenching them into your regular schedule.

So how does one define a habit? Habit is a continuously repeated behavior that we are often less conscious of. Most often than not, our environment triggers certain behaviors as an automatic response and requires no earlier intentions or preparations. According to a study, behavior becomes habitual once it is performed frequently or at least two times in a month and more extensively, up to ten times monthly, but it could take much longer than that.

An epidemiologist from the university college London, Philippa Lally researched to examine the formation of habits in our everyday life. This study was published in the European journal of social psychology in 2010. In her study, 22 adults were studied for 12 weeks and were asked to choose a healthy activity. Some chose to drink or eating behaviors that weren't part of their normal daily routine.

They were to perform these selected activities at the same time and place each day and were told to pen down a cue or situation that prompted such healthy activities as long as they continued to maintain them every day. She made sure not to include rewards of any kind as an incentive to encourage them to continue practicing such behavior.

The median length it took the participants to act automatically on such habits was 66 days. The range for the habit to be established was 18 to 254 days, but not all the subjects performed their chosen actions consistently as they should have. About half of the test subjects did not maintain their chosen habits consistently enough for it to become a habit. But one interesting fact Lally discovered is that increased repetition of an action does not always lead to strong habits.

She discovered that a habit could only be formed if a behavior is consistently repeated in the early process of habit formation. This way, behavior becomes more effective in creating an automatic action, and then repetition follows after later on. Furthermore, after a certain time, the process of habit-formation plateaus, so there is no further solidification of the repetition of the habit.

What her research suggests is that that it might take more days and weeks of diligence before a behavior becomes a habit, unlike the speculation that the habit-formation process usually 21 days. This shouldn't scare you but should help you recognize that behavior change could prove very challenging, especially dietary changes. Hence, you are encouraged to seek out ways to support your lifestyle tweaks.

Performing these new habits consistently and often would make them stick permanently into your daily routine. Developing healthy habits into our daily routine is all about preparing ourselves for success. When you have the right tools at your disposal, and you can keep yourself motivated, it is quite easy to make lifestyle changes and not as difficult as you think. So if you wish to develop healthy habits that will truly change your life, here are some helpful tools for you:

Create routines to make your mornings productive

Before you sleep at night, pick out your clothes and plan your breakfast so that your mornings roll by smoothly. We are not all aware of this, but research has shown that we are more productive during the mornings since we are still full of energy.

Read books that interest you

Whether it's a game of thrones novel or a suspenseful mystery such as gone girl, find something you're interested in as reading can help you build healthier habits. Reading books that keep your mind alert will help you be more productive throughout the day.

Pick a habit and keep track of your progress

Select a habit you wish to improve and then use a calendar or a habit-tracking app to keep track of your progress. Check off every day to ensure that you accomplish your task. If you happen to backslide on your task, there's no need to worry. Just take a breath and start again.

Make your workout routine slow but steady

While fitness is one of the most positive trends in the community, it can also put pressure on us to be healthy all the time. Don't push yourself to do too much. If you do, you might burn yourself out and even risk of injuries. Instead, find a workout you love and commit to doing it 2-3 times per week.

Select healthy foods you love genuinely

When you eat healthy foods that you genuinely love, you will find it very easy to eat healthily. Try out different healthy foods and find those that you genuinely love. Don't force yourself to eat whatever you don't like. You could browse healthy recipes that excite your taste buds.

What about eating out?

Going to a restaurant to eat out doesn't mean you should eat unhealthy foods. There are healthy meals that you can chew on at a restaurant. Follow these tips, and you will enjoy your meal, feel happy and satisfied when you're done.

Ask that your vegetables be doubled

Ask how the meal is prepared. Don't always go by the menu

Order from the healthy or light entrees

Avoid low-carb meal choices

Ask for double appetizers

Always order a salad first and watch out for unhealthy fats

Pay attention to add-ons on vegetable salads

Drink water before the meal

Skip the fancy drinks. Opt instead for a glass of wine, a light beer, a vodka, and tonic or a simple martini

Check the menu before you leave home

Skip the dessert, a small piece of chocolate should do

CONCLUSION

I hope you enjoyed reading this book as much as i loved writing it – and reading it too! It has been my pleasure writing to help those in need of guidance, and while. I would like to encourage you to practice what you read in this book from here on. I can guarantee that you will live healthier and feel better as long as you keep to the guidelines and tips in the book. I would also advise that constantly referring back to what you have read as well as getting additional information on the subject will help maintain a habit that will prove beneficial to your health in the long run.

If you ever feel confused about anything, you can always refer back to this book as I can assure you that that the information I provided will be your guide to total wholeness and a happy and healthy life – one that is leaky gut free. If you have any questions this book did not answer for you, please email them time at lauren@fixesfromnature.com, and I will make sure you have all the answers you need.

so in quick recaps, I'd like to go over some important points again so that you don't forget.

The leaky gut syndrome damages the lining of the intestines. It is a condition where gaps in the walls of the intestine allow bacteria and other toxins to enter the body's bloodstream. There is no need to panic because this condition can be improved. You just need to pay attention to some tiny details.

The small intestine breaks down food nutrients into small pieces that are easily absorbed by the body for energy, growth, and repair of body tissues. Our intestine helps to protect the body from harmful bacteria and toxins. The tight openings in the intestinal walls give room for water and nutrients to pass through and go into our bloodstream while also keeping aside harmful substances. When someone suffers from LGS, these intestinal openings become wider, which gives passage to food particles, bacteria, and toxins to enter our bloodstream directly.

There is a link between leaky gut syndrome and other health conditions like irritable bowel syndrome (IBS), Crohn's disease, celiac disease, chronic liver disease, diabetes, food allergies, and food sensitivities so if you suffer from LGS, it is possible that you're also suffering from the conditions mentioned above, but you should know that leaky gut is triggered by what we eat.

When you suffer from the leaky gut syndrome, you are every likely to experience one or more of these symptoms:

- Bloating
- Gas
- Cramps
- Food sensitivities
- Pin
- Autoimmune disease
- Thyroid problems
- Inflammatory skin conditions or acne

Several situations can trigger the symptoms of leaky gut ranging from poor diet to alcohol, inflammation, deficiency of vitamins, and so on. You should watch out for these risk factors in our everyday life to prevent the occurrence of other more severe infections and the effects of poor gut health. Some of the other conditions that could be triggered by a leaky gut are depression, eczema, rosacea, Alzheimer's disease, and many other horrible infections.

Since gut microbes affect brain health, changing gut bacteria is one of the reliable ways to improve brain health. Hence probiotics, live bacteria with so many benefits when it is consumed. However, they vary. Prebiotics are also helpful. They are mostly fibers that are fermented into the gut bacteria that also affect our brain's health. Probiotic supplements are also helpful; in the treatment of depressive symptoms as well as symptoms of depression, anxiety, obsessive-compulsive disorder, and other psychological and neurological conditions

One of the ways to living healthy and living a life free of leaky gut is to understand your body's healing ability and the one element that disrupts the body's healing ability - stress. Stressors damage the body's ability to heal itself. If we fail to put these stressors in check, our health will continue to deteriorate, causing us more pain, discomfort, and sometimes frustration.

The solution is to uncover the causes of these symptoms and decrease the stressors through appropriate treatment options, which will then allow the body to continue healing itself naturally, the leading cause of this infection is our diet, but diet does not mean losing weight or abstaining from certain kinds of food.

Diet refers to your overall eating habits, so diet means to eat, and I'm sure we all know that the moment we stop eating, we are less than a lifetime close to death. It is best to improve your actual diet and incorporate healthy changes to your lifestyle so that these changes eventually become a part of your normal lifestyle.

Most of these healthy diets incorporate mostly prebiotic and probiotic foods that support the growth and development of beneficial gut bacteria. Some of these foods include:

- Probiotic yogurt
- Roots and tubers
- Kefir or fermented yogurt
- Fermented foods
- Sourdough bread
- Some cheeses
- Vegetables
- Fruits
- Nuts and seeds
- Lactose-free dairy products
- Sprouted seeds
- Gluten-free grains
- Meat and eggs
- Herbs and spices
- Cultured dairy products
- Grains

Asides this information, the one true key to healing is our mindset, especially the growth mindset. People with growth mindsets are always constantly trying harder, trying everything possible to overcome the problem or situation they find themselves. With this mindset, you will be energized and encouraged to follow the principles and tips to heal your gut as well as make your life healthier.

Finally, you have to develop healthy habits for a healthy life. Some certain habits are dangerous to our health, and until we switch to a healthy lifestyle, we cannot possibly maintain our health. Developing healthy habits into our daily routine is all about preparing ourselves for success. It is possible that in some people, certain foods are more likely to trigger symptoms more than other kinds of food. It could be helpful to use a food journal to keep track of one's dietary habits as well as the symptoms they experience and to point out the trigger foods that trigger their symptoms.

Breakfast Recipes

Gut-Healing Smoothie

Aloe-Mint Smoothie

Cinnamon Berry Smoothie

Spinach and Aloe Smoothie

Berry Flax Smoothie

Strawberry Healthy Gut Smoothie

Apple-Banana Smoothie

Turmeric Latte

Herb Scrambled Egg with Asparagus

Sausage and Sauerkraut

Banana, Flax and Turmeric Oats

Sweet Miso Porridge

Buckwheat Pancakes

Lemony Quinoa

Lunch Recipes

Beef and Veggie Burgers

Turmeric Cauliflower Soup

Chicken Pesto Pasta with Asparagus

Tomato-less Soup

Herb Bone Marrow

Smoked Salmon with Spinach and Lemon Salad

Baked Chicken

Grilled Sauerkraut Avocado Sandwich

Garlic Shrimp in Butter Sauce

Mushroom and Leek Soup

Chicken Meatballs with Greens

<u>Veggie Stir Fry</u>

<u>Roasted Broccoli</u>

Dinner Recipes

<u>Veggies and Shrimp with Rice Noodles</u>

<u>Chicken Thighs with Pineapple Salsa</u>

<u>Salmon with Green Beans</u>

<u>Chicken Piccata</u>

<u>Creamy Potato and Chicken Soup</u>

<u>Superfood Burger</u>

<u>Taco Soup</u>

<u>Thai Chickpea Curry</u>

<u>Turkey Soup</u>

<u>BBQ Tempeh Wrap</u>

<u>Coconut Chicken Curry</u>

<u>Veggie Packed Soup</u>

<u>Beef Ragu with Spaghetti Squash</u>

<u>Almond-Crusted Cod with Greens</u>

Desserts

<u>Banana and Mint Chip Ice Cream</u>

<u>Baked Stuffed Apples</u>

<u>Poached Pears</u>

<u>Mango and Lime Sorbet</u>

Salads

<u>Lentil and Squash Salad</u>

<u>Sauerkraut Salad</u>

<u>Avocado and Papaya Salad</u>

<u>Mango and Red Cabbage Salad</u>

<u>Roasted Veggie Salad</u>

<u>Soups</u>

<u>Chicken and Chickpea Soup</u>

<u>Chicken Zoodle Pho</u>

<u>Mexicali Chicken Soup</u>

<u>Emerald City Soup</u>

<u>Butternut Squash Soup</u>

Breakfast Recipes

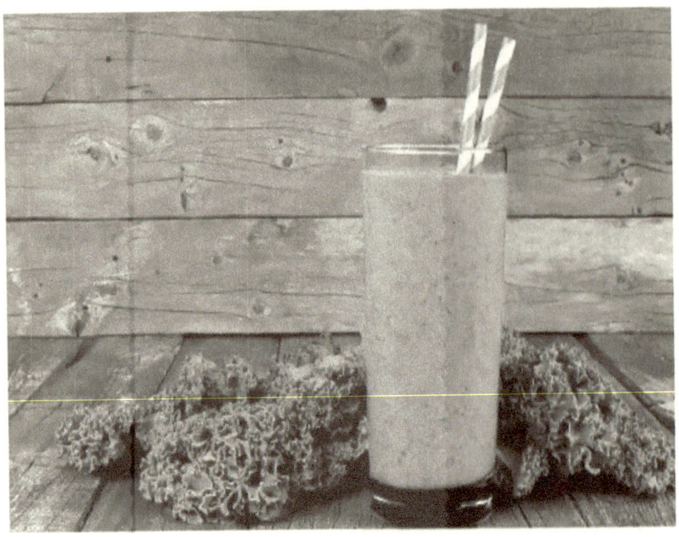

Serves: 4 smoothie glasses; Prep time: 5 minutes; Cooking time: 0 minutes; Total time: 5 minutes;

Nutritional values per serving:

Calories: 112.5 Cal; Fat: 8.4 g; Carbs: 4.8 g; Protein: 4.5 g; Fiber: 1.5 g;

Ingredients:

- 4 cups chopped organic kale
- 1 cup of organic mixed berries, frozen
- 1 teaspoon probiotic powder

- 2 teaspoons zinc carnosine
- 4 tablespoons grass-fed collagen protein powder
- 2 teaspoons deglycyrrhizinated licorice (DGL)
- 2 tablespoons coconut oil
- 2 tablespoons L-glutamine powder
- 2 cups almond milk, unsweetened

Instructions:

- Take a blender, add all the ingredients for smoothie in it, and pulse for 1 to 2 minutes until smooth.
- Evenly divide the smoothie between four glasses and serve.

Aloe-Mint Smoothie

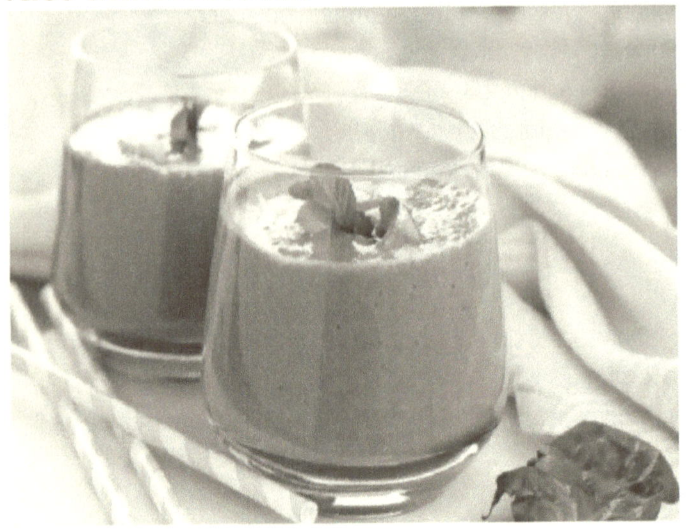

Serves: 4 smoothie glasses; Prep time: 5 minutes; Cooking time: 0 minutes; Total time: 5 minutes;

Nutritional values per serving:

Calories: 337 Cal; Fat: 20.6 g; Carbs: 17 g; Protein: 21.1 g; Fiber: 7.1 g;

Ingredients:

- 1 cup organic blueberries, frozen
- 2 tablespoons chia seeds
- 1/2 inch of organic ginger root
- 1 medium organic avocado, peeled, pitted, diced
- ¼ cup mint leaves
- 6 tablespoons collagen hydrolysate
- 4 tablespoons coconut oil

- 8 fluid ounces aloe vera juice
- 2 cups of coconut water

Instructions:

- Take a blender, add all the ingredients for smoothie in it, and pulse for 1 to 2 minutes until smooth.
- Evenly divide the smoothie between four glasses and serve.

Cinnamon Berry Smoothie

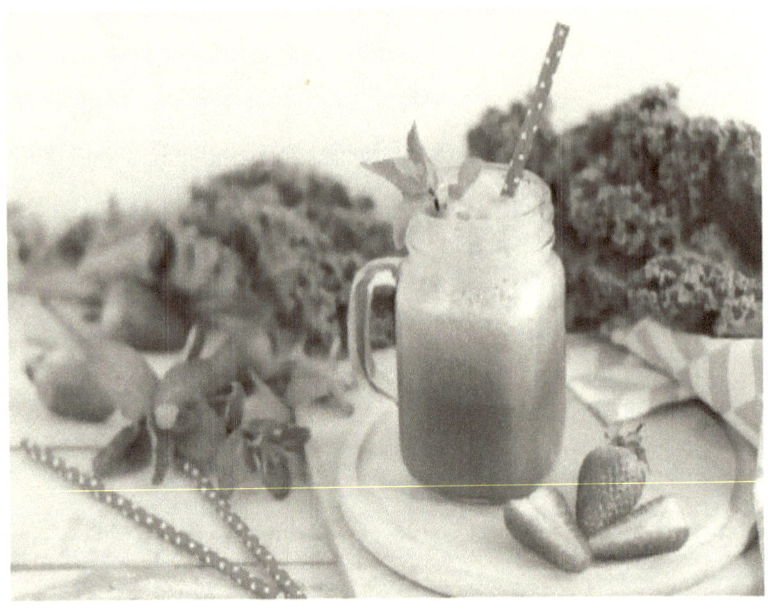

Serves: 4 smoothie glasses; Prep time: 5 minutes; Cooking time: 0 minutes; Total time: 5 minutes;

Nutritional values per serving:

Calories: 113.5 Cal; Fat: 7.2 g; Carbs: 9.9 g; Protein: 2.3 g; Fiber: 4.3 g;

Ingredients:

- 2 cups organic strawberries, frozen
- 2 cups organic kale
- ½ teaspoon cinnamon
- 1 medium organic avocado, pitted

- 10 drops vanilla extract, unsweetened
- 3 cups almond milk, unsweetened

Instructions:

- Take a blender, add all the ingredients for smoothie in it, and pulse for 1 to 2 minutes until smooth.
- Evenly divide the smoothie between four glasses and serve.

Spinach and Aloe Smoothie

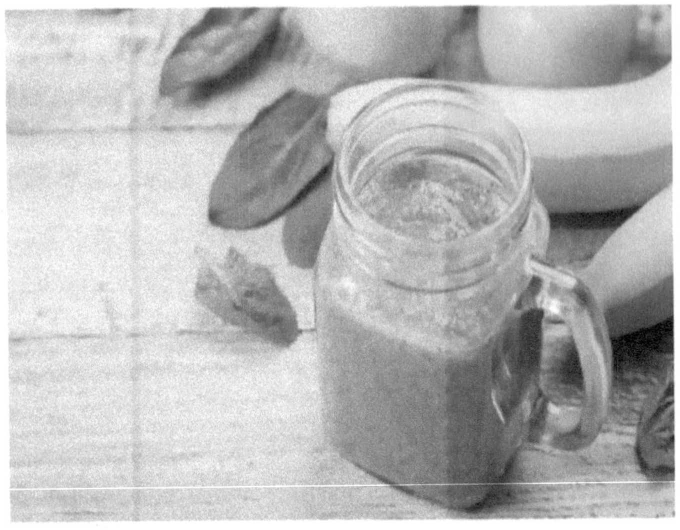

Serves: 4 smoothie glasses; **Prep time:** 5 minutes; Cooking time: 0 minutes; Total time: 5 minutes;

Nutritional values per serving:

Calories: 108 Cal; Fat: 2 g; Carbs: 8.6 g; Protein: 13.8 g; Fiber: 2.1 g;

Ingredients:

- 4 cups fresh organic spinach
- 4 teaspoons vanilla extract, unsweetened
- 4 teaspoons cinnamon
- 2 cups Greek yogurt
- 4 fluid ounces aloe vera juice

- 2 cups almond milk, unsweetened

Instructions:

- Take a blender, add all the ingredients for smoothie in it, and pulse for 1 to 2 minutes until smooth.
- Evenly divide the smoothie between four glasses and serve.

Berry Flax Smoothie

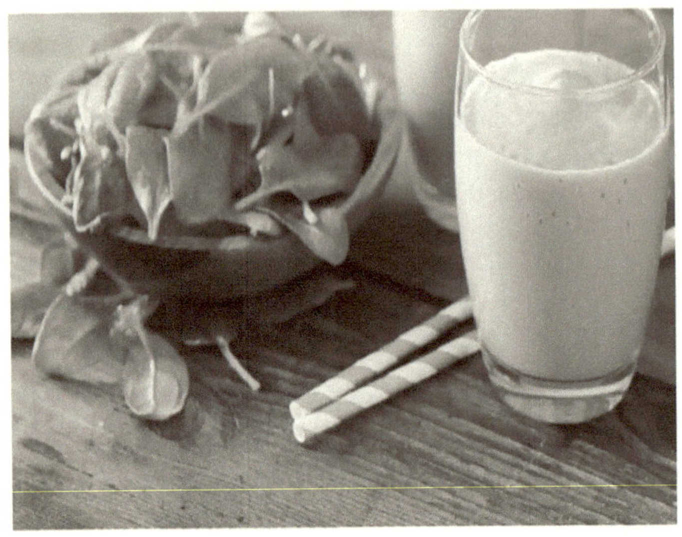

Serves: 4 smoothie glasses; Prep time: 5 minutes; Cooking time: 0 minutes; Total time: 5 minutes;

Nutritional values per serving:

Calories: 82 Cal; Fat: 4.4 g; Carbs: 8.2 g; Protein: 2.5 g; Fiber: 2.6 g;

Ingredients:

- 2 cups fresh organic spinach
- 2 tablespoons flax seeds, ground
- ½ cup of organic strawberries, frozen
- ½ cup organic blueberries, frozen
- 2 teaspoons grated organic ginger

- 4 cups almond milk, unsweetened

Instructions:

- Take a blender, add all the ingredients for smoothie in it, and pulse for 1 to 2 minutes until smooth.
- Evenly divide the smoothie between four glasses and serve.

Strawberry Healthy Gut Smoothie

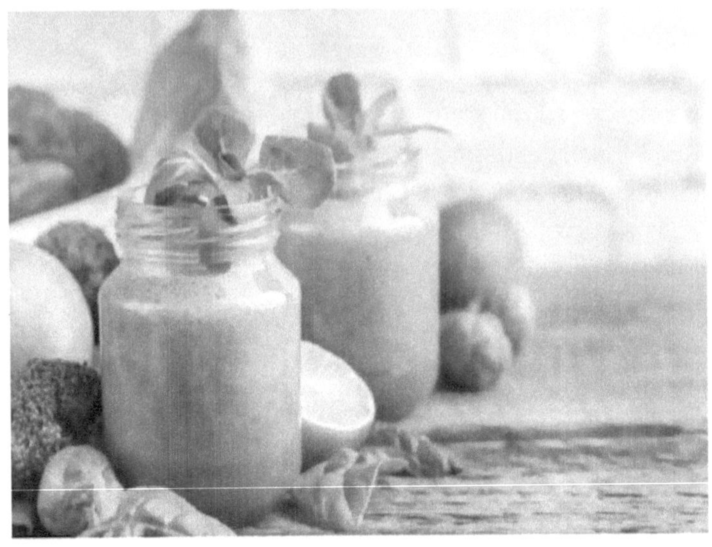

Serves: 4 smoothie glasses; Prep time: 5 minutes; Cooking time: 0 minutes; Total time: 5 minutes;

Nutritional values per serving:

Calories: 111.8 Cal; Fat: 5.5 g; Carbs: 13.4 g; Protein: 2.2 g; Fiber: 6 g;

Ingredients:

- 2 cups organic romaine lettuce
- 1 cup organic strawberries, frozen
- 1 medium organic avocado, peeled, pitted, diced
- 2 cups organic kale
- 3 cups of coconut water

Instructions:

- Take a blender, add all the ingredients for smoothie in it, and pulse for 1 to 2 minutes until smooth.
- Evenly divide the smoothie between four glasses and serve.

Apple-Banana Smoothie

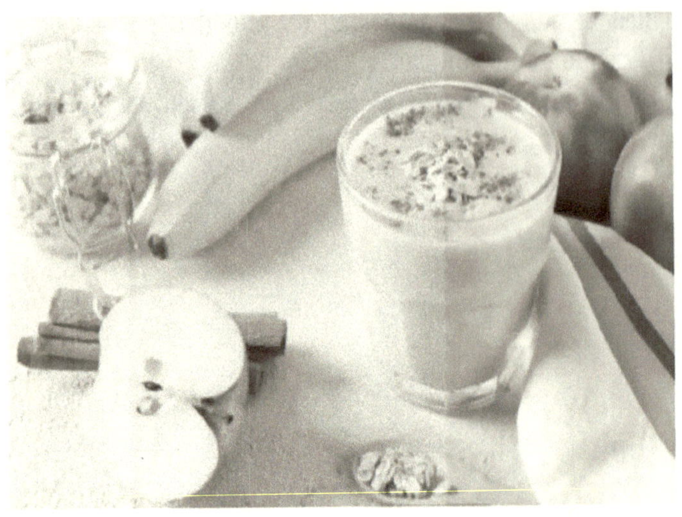

Serves: 4 smoothie glasses; Prep time: 5 minutes;
Cooking time: 0 minutes; Total time: 5 minutes;

Nutritional values per serving:

Calories: 389.3 Cal; Fat: 16.4 g; Carbs: 37 g; Protein:
23.4 g; Fiber: 8.5 g;

Ingredients:

- 20 walnuts
- 2 medium organic apple, cored, chopped
- 4 tablespoons chia seeds
- 2 medium organic banana, peeled, sliced
- 2 teaspoons cinnamon
- 3 cups Greek yogurt

- 2 cups of ice cubes
- 1 cup of water

Instructions:

- Take a blender, add all the ingredients for smoothie in it, and pulse for 1 to 2 minutes until smooth.
- Evenly divide the smoothie between four glasses, sprinkle with additional cinnamon and serve.

Turmeric Latte

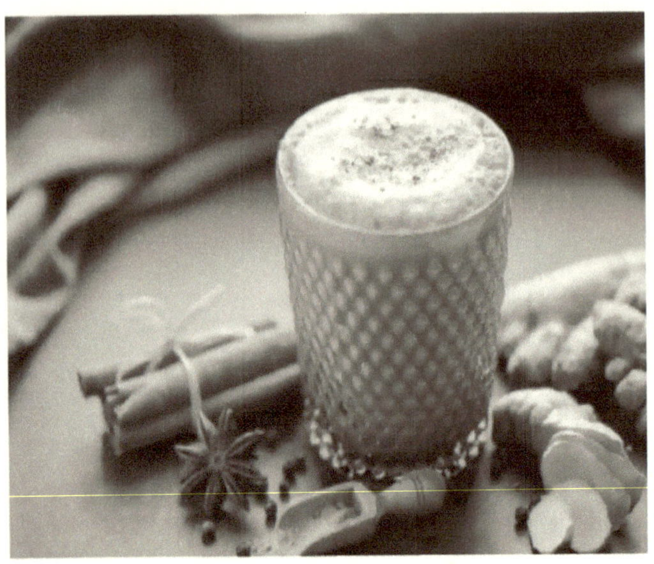

Serves: 4 glasses; Prep time: 5 minutes; Cooking time: 0 minutes; Total time: 5 minutes;

Nutritional values per serving:

Calories: 62.8 Cal; Fat: 4.3 g; Carbs: 5.5 g; Protein: 0.6 g; Fiber: 1.4 g;

Ingredients:

- 2-inch fresh organic ginger root, peeled, chopped
- 2 teaspoons ground turmeric
- 2 teaspoons ground cinnamon
- 2 teaspoons raw honey
- 4 cups coconut milk, unsweetened

Instructions:

- Take a blender, add all the ingredients for smoothie in it, and pulse for 1 to 2 minutes until smooth.
- Evenly divide the smoothie between four glasses and serve.

Herb Scrambled Egg with Asparagus

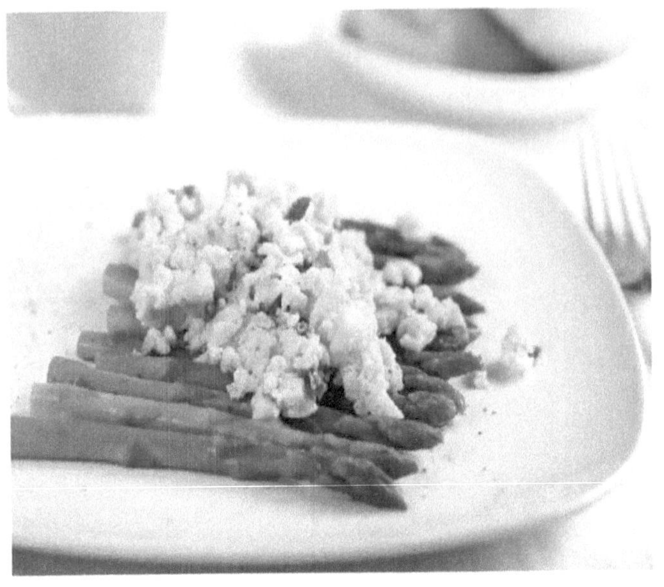

Serves: 4 plates; Prep time: 5 minutes; Cooking time: 10 minutes; Total time: 15 minutes;

Nutritional values per serving:

Calories: 210 Cal; Fat: 14 g; Carbs: 1 g; Protein: 21 g; Fiber: 0 g;

Ingredients:

- 7 ounces organic asparagus spears, peeled, scaled
- ½ cup chopped organic tarragon
- ½ teaspoon salt
- ½ teaspoon ground black pepper

- 4 tablespoons unsalted butter
- 8 pasteurized eggs
- Grated cottage cheese, for topping
- Slices of sourdough bread, toasted
- ½ cup of water

Instructions:

- Rinse the asparagus thoroughly, then peel and scale them and cut into bite-size pieces.
- Take an ovenproof casserole dish, pour in water, add asparagus in layers, and cover the top with a plastic wrap.
- Make holes in the plastic wrap by poking fork in it and then microwave asparagus for 4 to 5 minutes until done, checking asparagus every 2 minutes.
- When done, remove the casserole dish from the oven, remove the plastic wrap, transfer asparagus to a plate, and set aside until required.
- Prepare the scrambled eggs and for this, take a large skillet pan, add butter and let it melt until it starts to melts.
- Crack the eggs in a bowl, whisk until blended, then pour the eggs into the pan and cook the eggs until scrambled to desire level.
- Season eggs with salt and black pepper, add tarragon, stir well and remove the pan from heat.
- Evenly divide asparagus between four plates, top them evenly with scrambled eggs, sprinkle with cheese, and serve with a toast of sourdough bread.

Sausage and Sauerkraut

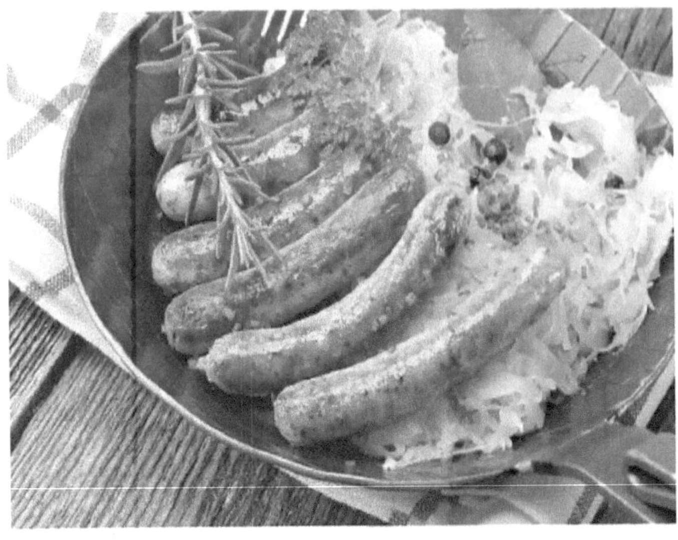

Serves: 4 plates; Prep time: 5 minutes; Cooking time: 20 minutes; Total time: 25 minutes;

Nutritional values per serving:

Calories: 351.5 Cal; Fat: 23 g; Carbs: 26.4 g; Protein: 9.7 g; Fiber: 9.8 g;

Ingredients:

- 8 grass-fed beef sausages, uncured
- 2 medium organic white onion, peeled, sliced
- 2 medium organic apples, cored, sliced
- 4 cups organic sauerkraut
- 1 teaspoon ground black pepper

- ½ teaspoon caraway seeds
- 4 tablespoons unsalted butter
- 1 cup sauerkraut liquid

Instructions:

- Take a large skillet pan, place it over medium-low heat, add butter and when it melts, add onions and cook for 5 minutes until softened.
- Switch heat to the low level, sprinkle black pepper and caraway seeds over onions, add sauerkraut, pour in sauerkraut liquid, stir until mixed and simmer for 20 minutes, covering the pan.
- Meanwhile, take a grilling pan, place it over medium heat, grease it with coconut oil and when hot, add sausages and cook for 15 to 20 minutes until thoroughly cooked, turning every 5 minutes.
- When sausages have cooked, let them rest for 5 minutes and then divide them into four plates, two sausages per plate.
- Add sauerkraut mixture, then add some apple slices and serve.

Banana, Flax and Turmeric Oats

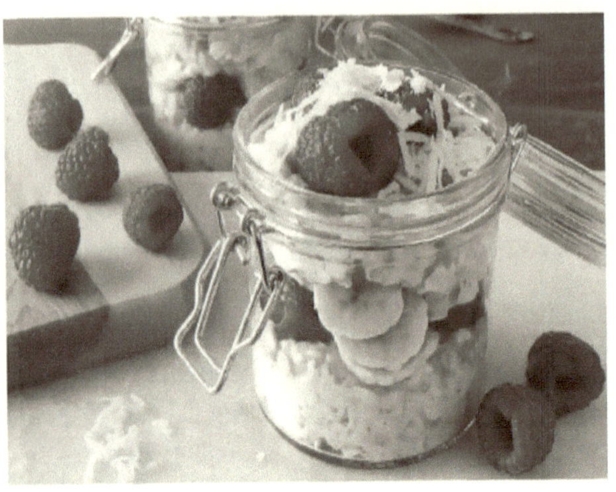

Serves: 4 bowls; Prep time: 4 hours and 5 minutes; Cooking time: 0 minutes; Total time: 4 hours and 5 minutes;

Nutritional values per serving:

Calories: 419.3 Cal; Fat: 16.3 g; Carbs: 58.7 g; Protein: 9.4 g; Fiber: 12.3 g;

Ingredients:

- ½ cup ground flaxseed
- 4 small organic bananas, peeled
- 2 cups rolled oats
- 4 teaspoons ground turmeric
- 2 teaspoons ground cinnamon
- 2 cups almond milk, unsweetened

- ½ cup Greek yogurt
- 2 cups of water
- Raspberries for serving

Instructions:

- Take a jar or container, add flaxseeds, oats, turmeric, and cinnamon and stir until mixed.
- Place bananas in a shallow dish, mash well with a fork and then add to the oats mixture.
- Add yogurt, pour in water and milk, stir until well combined, pour the mixture over fruits and oats and refrigerate for a minimum of 4 hours or overnight.
- When ready to eat, evenly divide them between four bowls, top with berries or any other favorite toppings and serve.

Sweet Miso Porridge

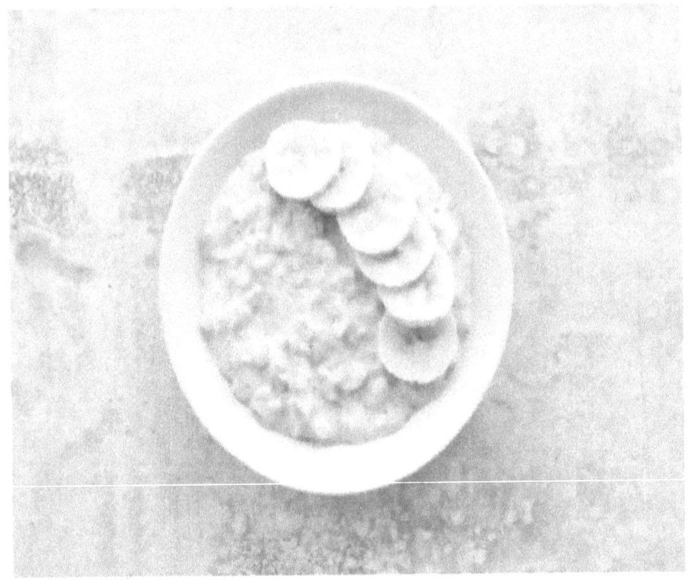

Serves: 4 bowls; Prep time: 10 minutes; Cooking time: 10 minutes; Total time: 20 minutes;

Nutritional values per serving:

Calories: 1285 Cal; Fat: 31.4 g; Carbs: 221.7 g; Protein: 29 g; Fiber: 30 g;

Ingredients:

For Porridge:

- 4 cups rolled porridge oats
- 1/2 teaspoons ground ginger
- 1 tablespoon chia seeds

- 1 tablespoon white sweet miso
- 1/2 teaspoon vanilla powder
- 2 cardamom pods
- 8 cups almond milk

For Topping:

- 4 medium organic banana, peeled, sliced
- 4 medium organic pears, diced
- ½ cup pecan nuts
- 4 tablespoons raw honey

Instructions:

- Prepare the porridge and for this, take a medium saucepan, place it over medium-high heat, add chia seeds, oats, and ginger and pour in the milk.
- Crush the seeds of cardamom, add to the porridge, stir well and cook for 8 to 10 minutes until oats have cooked, and most of the liquid is absorbed.
- Remove pan from heat, add vanilla powder and miso paste, stir well and then evenly divide porridge between four bowls.
- Top evenly with banana, pear, nuts, and honey and serve straight away.

Buckwheat Pancakes

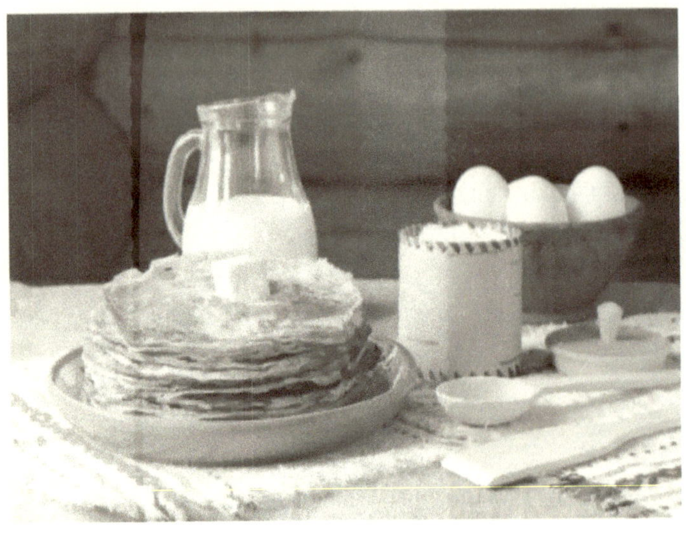

Serves: 4; Prep time: 10 minutes; Cooking time: 30 minutes; Total time: 40 minutes;

Nutritional values per serving:

Calories: 107 Cal; Fat: 102 g; Carbs: 21 g; Protein: 3 g; Fiber: 3 g;

Ingredients:

- 1 cup buckwheat flour
- 1 1/2 cup mashed organic banana
- 2 teaspoons ground cinnamon
- 2 teaspoons baking soda
- 4 teaspoons apple cider vinegar
- 2 teaspoons vanilla extract, unsweetened

- 4 tablespoons coconut oil
- 4 tablespoons water

Instructions:

- Take a medium bowl, add mashed bananas in it along with remaining ingredients and stir well until smooth and thick batter comes together.
- Take a medium skillet pan, place it over medium heat, grease the pan with oil, and when hot, pour in ¼ cup of batter, spread it evenly with a back of a spoon to create a 1/4-inch thick pancake and cook for 4 to 5 minutes per side until nicely golden.
- Cook more pancakes using the remaining batter and serve with fresh fruits and honey.

- ***Buckwheat Bread***

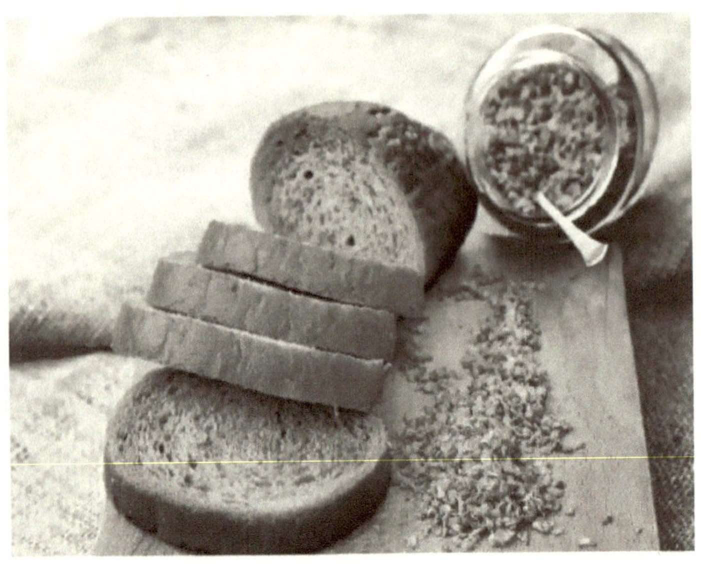

Serves: 1 small loaf; Prep time: 1 hour and 10 minutes; Cooking time: 1 hour and 10 minutes; Total time: 2 hours and 20 minutes;

Nutritional values per serving:

Calories: 600 Cal; Fat: 0 g; Carbs: 120 g; Protein: 18 g; Fiber: 12 g;

Ingredients:

- 1 cup buckwheat flour
- 3 tablespoons psyllium husk
- 1 1/2 cups almond meal

- 1/2 teaspoon salt
- 2 tablespoons raw honey
- 2 teaspoons bicarb soda
- 3 tablespoons chia seeds
- 1/3 cup buckwheat groats
- 1/3 cup sunflower seeds
- 1/3 cup pumpkin seeds
- 2 tablespoons apple cider vinegar
- 2 cups of water
- Scrambled eggs for serving

Instructions:

- Take a medium bowl, pour in water, add vinegar and honey and whisk well until combined.
- Take a large bowl, add buckwheat flour along with remaining ingredients, stir well, then make a well in the center of bowl, pour vinegar mixture in it and mix until thoroughly combined.
- Cover the bowl containing dough with a tea towel and let it rest for 1 hour at a warm place.
- In the meantime, switch on the oven, then set it to 350 degrees F, and let it preheat.
- After 1 hour, transfer the dough into a greased 8-by-4 inches loaf pan, smooth the top and bake for 1 hour and 10 minutes until the top has turned very dark brown and bread is very firm to touch.
- When done, let the bread cool in the pan for 15 minutes, then take out the bread and cool it completely on a wire rack.
- Slice the bread and serve it with scrambled eggs or eat it as you want.

Lemony Quinoa

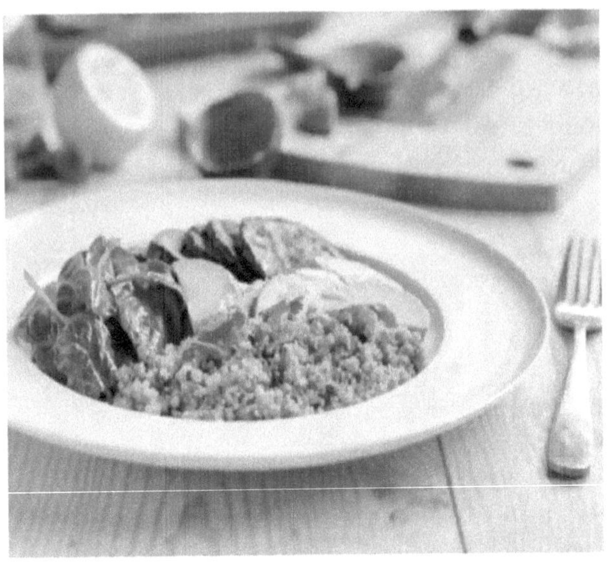

Serves: 4; Prep time: 5 minutes; Cooking time: 25 minutes; Total time: 30 minutes;

Nutritional values per serving:

Calories: 439.8 Cal; Fat: 22 g; Carbs: 46.2 g; Protein: 14.3 g; Fiber: 7 g;

Ingredients:

- 1 cup uncooked quinoa, rinsed, drained
- 3/4 cup fresh cilantro
- 3/4 cup toasted almonds, chopped
- 1/2 cup organic raisins
- 1/2 teaspoon cumin powder

- 1 teaspoon turmeric powder
- 1 teaspoon curry powder
- 2 tablespoons olive oil
- 2 cups of chicken bone broth
- 1/2 of a lemon, juiced

Instructions:

- Take a medium saucepan, place it over medium-low heat, add oil and when hot, add cumin powder, turmeric powder, curry powder, stir well and cook for 2 minutes until fragrant.
- Then switch the heat to medium-low level, add quinoa in the pan and cook for 3 minutes until sizzles, stirring continuously.
- Switch heat to the low level, pour in chicken broth, mix it well and simmer quinoa for 20 minutes until the quinoa has cooked, covering the pan.
- Then remove the pan from heat, let quinoa sit for 5 minutes and then fluff with a fork.
- Transfer quinoa to a large bowl, add remaining ingredients, toss until well mixed and serve.

Lunch Recipes

Beef and Veggie Burgers

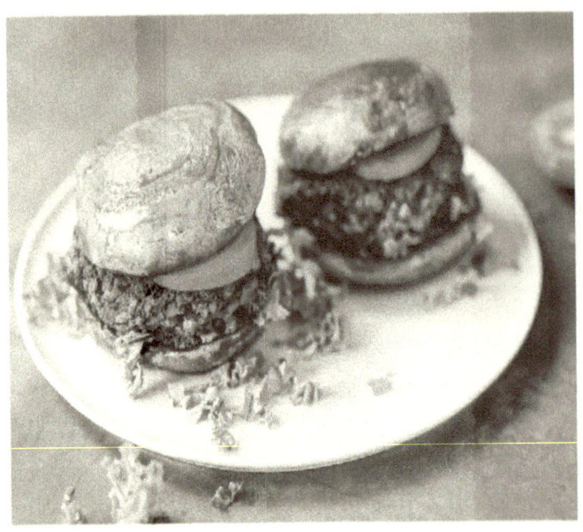

Serves: 4 burgers; Prep time: 10 minutes; Cooking time: 30 minutes; Total time: 40 minutes;

Nutritional values per serving:

Calories: 453.8 Cal; Fat: 29.2 g; Carbs: 14.7 g; Protein: 33 g; Fiber: 5 g;

Ingredients:

For Patties:

- 1 medium organic carrots, peeled, grated
- 1 pound grass-fed ground beef
- 1 medium organic zucchini, grated

- 2 tablespoons chopped fresh parsley
- 1 teaspoon minced organic garlic
- ¼ teaspoon salt
- ¼ teaspoon ground black pepper
- 1 tablespoon grated parmesan cheese
- 1 ½ tablespoon coconut oil

For Burger:

- 1 large organic sweet potato, peeled
- 4 large leaves of organic lettuce
- 4 slices of organic tomato
- 4 slices of organic avocado

Instructions:

- Prepare the patties and for this, take a medium skillet pan, place it over medium heat, add ¾ tablespoon oil and when it melts, add grated carrot and zucchini, add garlic, season with salt and black pepper, stir well and cook for 3 minutes.
- Then add parsley, stir until mixed and cook for 3 to 5 minutes or until vegetables have softened.
- Remove pan from heat, transfer vegetables to a bowl, and let it cool enough to be handled by hands.
- Add beef and parmesan cheese to the vegetables, mix well until combined, and then shape the mixture into four patties.
- Return the skillet pan over medium-high heat, add remaining oil and when it melts, add prepared patties in it and cook for 3 to 4 minutes per side until browned.
- To assemble the burger, microwave the sweet potato for 2 minutes and then cut it into ¼-inch thick rounds.
- Take a griddle pan, place it over medium-high heat, grease it with oil, add sweet potatoes slices, and grill for 5 to 6 minutes per side until done.
- Working on one burger at a time, take a grilled slice of sweet

potato, line it with a lettuce leaf, then top with a patty, an avocado slice, and a tomato slice, and cover with another slice of sweet potato.

- Prepare three more burgers in the same manner and serve straight away.

Turmeric Cauliflower Soup

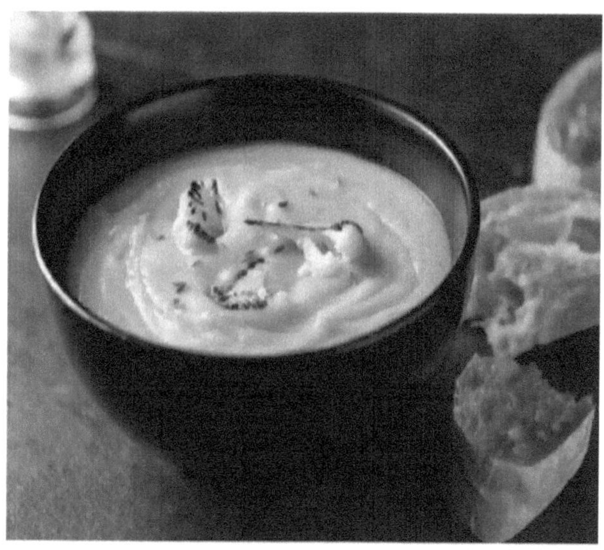

Serves: 4 bowls; Prep time: 10 minutes; Cooking time: 50 minutes; Total time: 60 minutes;

Nutritional values per serving:

Calories: 187 Cal; Fat: 9 g; Carbs: 19 g; Protein: 7 g; Fiber: 8 g;

Ingredients:

- 1 medium head of organic cauliflower, chopped
- 1 medium organic shallot, quartered
- 1/2 cup red lentils
- 4 cloves of garlic, peeled
- 1/2 teaspoon sea salt

- 1 teaspoon cracked black pepper
- 1 teaspoon ground turmeric
- 1 teaspoon ground cumin
- 2 tablespoons olive oil and more for topping
- 2 1/2 cups almond milk and cashew milk blend, divided
- 2 cups vegetable broth
- 4 teaspoon chopped chives

Instructions:

- Switch on the oven, then set it to 425 degrees F and let it preheat.
- Meanwhile, place cauliflower florets in a bowl, add shallots pieces and garlic cloves, drizzle with oil, season with salt, black pepper, cumin, and turmeric and toss until well coated.
- Take a baking sheet, transfer vegetables on it, spread them evenly and roast for 30 minutes, flipping the vegetables halfway through.
- When done, transfer roasted vegetables to a saucepan, add lentil, pour in vegetable broth, and 2 cups of milk blend, stir well and bring it to boil over medium-low heat.
- Then lower heat to medium-low level and simmer the soup for 20 minutes, covering the pan.
- After 20 minutes, remove the pan from heat, puree the soup by using an immersion blender until smooth, pour in remaining milk and stir until well mixed.
- Ladle soup into four bowls, top with chives, drizzle with some olive oil and serve.

Chicken Pesto Pasta with Asparagus

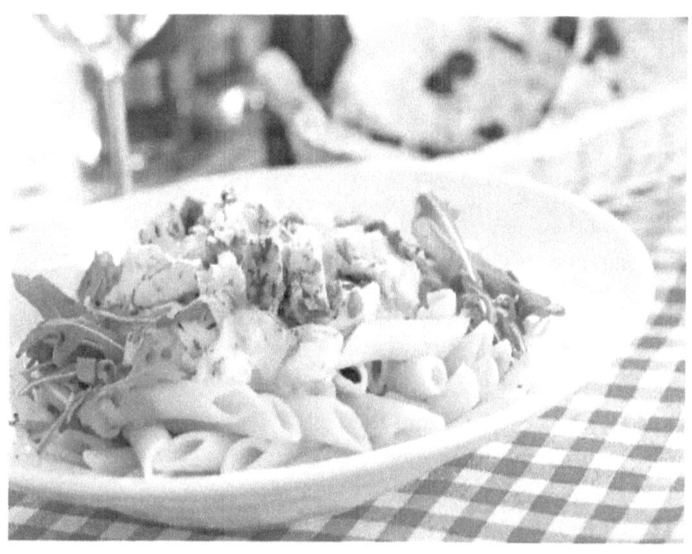

Serves: 4; Prep time: 10 minutes; Cooking time: 10 minutes; Total time: 20 minutes;

Nutritional values per serving:

Calories: 422 Cal; Fat: 18 g; Carbs: 32 g; Protein: 31 g; Fiber: 1 g;

Ingredients:

- 2 cups shredded cooked antibiotic-free, pasteurized chicken breast
- 6 ounces whole-wheat penne pasta
- ¾ pound fresh organic asparagus, trimmed, peeled, scaled, cut into 2-inch pieces
- ¾ teaspoon salt
- ¼ teaspoon ground black pepper
- 4 ounces organic basil pesto
- 2 tablespoons grated parmesan cheese

- Basil leaves for garnish

Instructions:

- Place a medium pot half-full with salted water over medium heat, add pasta and cook for 7 to 10 minutes until tender.
- Add asparagus pieces during the last two minutes of pasta cooking time, and then drain the pasta and asparagus, reserving ½ cup of cooking liquid.
- Return pasta and asparagus into the pan, add chicken and pesto, season with salt and black pepper and stir in the reserved cooking liquid, 1 tablespoon at a time until pasta reached to desired consistency.
- Distribute the pasta evenly between four plates, garnish with parmesan cheese and basil leaves and serve straight away.

Tomato-less Soup

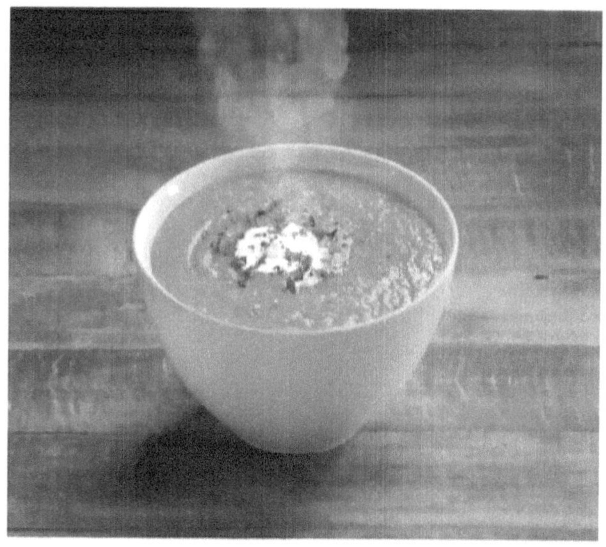

Serves: 4; Prep time: 10 minutes; Cooking time: 50 minutes; Total time: 60 minutes;

Nutritional values per serving:

Calories: 233 Cal; Fat: 11 g; Carbs: 25 g; Protein: 8.7 g; Fiber: 6.6 g;

Ingredients:

- 1 pound fresh organic beets, scrubbed, top removed
- 8 ounces organic carrots, peeled, chopped
- 1 medium organic white onion , peeled, chopped
- 1 cup chopped organic celery
- 2 teaspoons sea salt

- 1 teaspoon dried savory
- 2 tablespoons coconut oil
- 6 tablespoons apple cider vinegar
- 6 tablespoons lemon juice
- 14 ounces pumpkin puree
- 4 cups of chicken bone broth
- 3 tablespoons chopped parsley

Instructions:

- Take a small saucepan, add beets in it, then pour in enough water to cover them, and bring the beets to boil over medium-high heat.
- Then lower heat to medium-low level and simmer the beets for 20 to 25 minutes until beets are tender and cooking liquid has turned into ruby red color.
- When done, drain the beets and set aside until required.
- Take a large pot, place it over medium-low heat, add oil and when it melts, add celery, onion, and carrots and cook for 7 to 10 minutes until sautéed.
- Then increase heat to medium-high level, add beets into the pot, pour in pumpkin puree and chicken broth, stir well and bring the mixture to boil.
- Lower heat to medium-low level and simmer the vegetables for 10 to 15 minutes until softened.
- Then remove the pot from heat and puree the vegetables by using an immersion blender until smooth.
- Stir in vinegar and lemon juice, one tablespoon at a time, and testing the soup, until soup has reached to desired taste.
- Stir in salt and savory, taste the soup to adjust seasoning and then ladle soup into four bowls.
- Garnish soup with parsley and serve.

Herb Bone Marrow

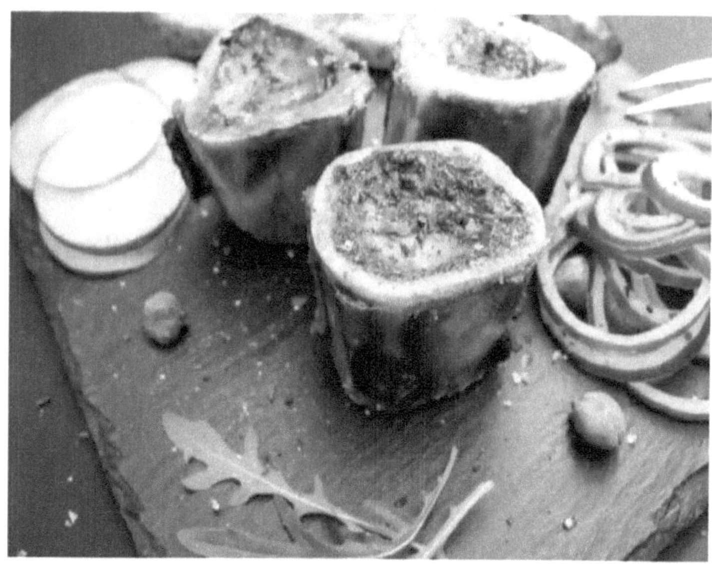

Serves: 4; Prep time: 5 minutes; Cooking time: 15 minutes; Total time: 20 minutes;

Nutritional values per serving:

Calories: 104 Cal; Fat: 11 g; Carbs: 0 g; Protein: 1 g; Fiber: 0 g;

Ingredients:

- 8 frozen grass-fed beef marrow bones, thawed
- 1 teaspoon salt
- 1 teaspoon ground black pepper
- 1 teaspoon chopped fresh organic rosemary
- 1 teaspoon chopped fresh organic thyme

Instructions:

- Switch on the oven, then set it to 425 degrees F and let it preheat.
- Then place bone marrow in a baking dish, sprinkle with rosemary and thyme, and roast for 15 minutes until marrows are no longer from inside.
- When done, remove the baking dish from the oven and season marrows with salt and black pepper.
- Serve straight away and have it by scooping out the marrow from the bone.

Smoked Salmon with Spinach and Lemon Salad

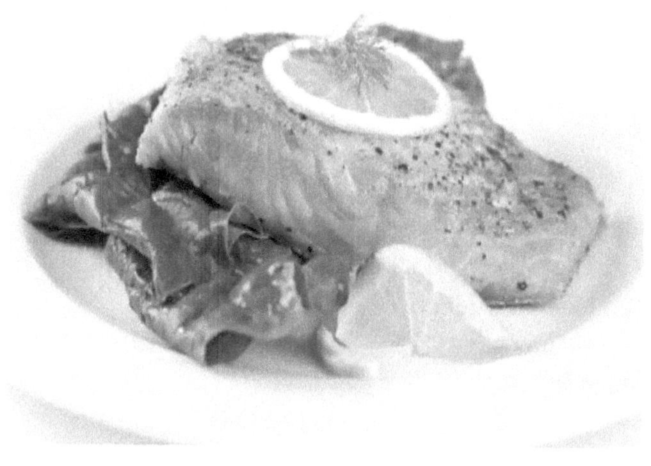

Serves: 4; Prep time: 10 minutes; Cooking time: 5 minutes; Total time: 15 minutes;

Nutritional values per serving:

Calories: 106 Cal; Fat: 5.4 g; Carbs: 2.2 g; Protein: 12.2 g; Fiber: 1.2 g;

Ingredients:

- 4 pieces of hot smoked wild-caught salmon, each about 4-ounce
- 3 cups fresh organic spinach
- 2 organic lemons
- ¾ teaspoon ground black pepper
- 1 teaspoon salt
- 4 teaspoons capers

- 4 teaspoons caster sugar
- 4 tablespoons olive oil

Instructions:

- Peel the lemon, cut it into thin slices, and add it in a bowl along with its juice.
- Add capers, sugar, and oil and stir until well mixed.
- Steam the spinach and for this, place a medium pot half full with water over medium heat, bring the water to boil, then add spinach and steam for 1 minute until the leaf begins to wilt.
- Plunge the steamed spinach immediately into cold, then drain it well and transfer to a plate.
- Evenly divide spinach between four plates, then top with salmon, add lemon mixture and serve.

Baked Chicken

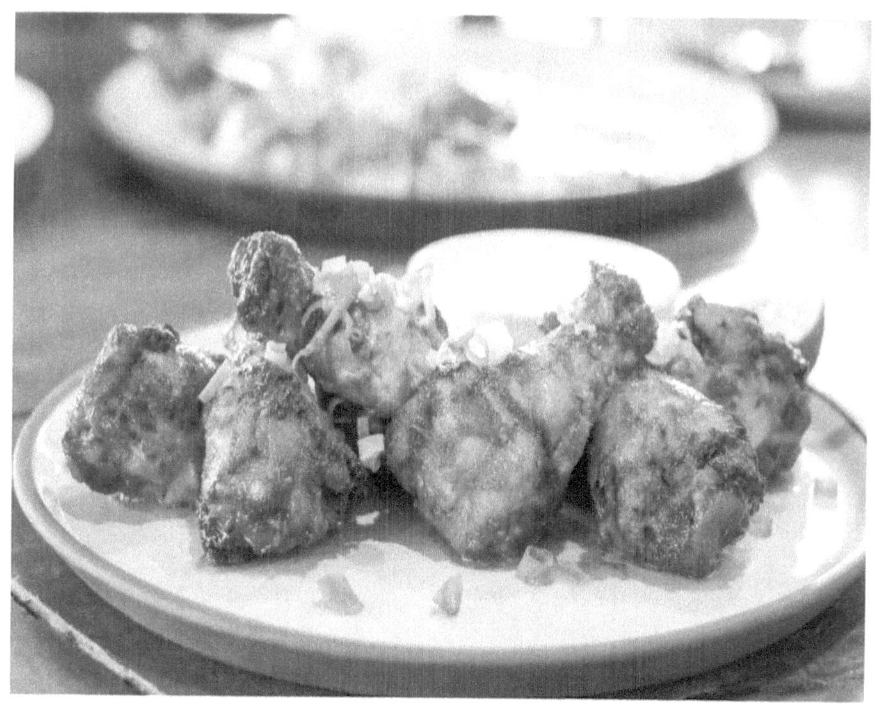

Serves: 4; Prep time: 10 minutes; Cooking time: 1 hour; Total time: 1 hour and 10 minutes;

Nutritional values per serving:

Calories: 353.8 Cal; Fat: 13.8 g; Carbs: 26.5 g; Protein: 31 g; Fiber: 9.9 g;

Ingredients:

- 4 large antibiotic-free, pasteurized, pasteurized chicken thighs,

boneless, skinless
- 1 small organic fennel bulb, trimmed, cut in eighths lengthwise
- 16 organic cherry tomatoes
- 8 ounces organic green beans
- 1 medium organic red bell pepper, deseeded, cut into strip
- 1 teaspoon paprika
- 1 ½ teaspoon ground black pepper
- 2 teaspoons sea salt
- 1 tablespoon chopped organic tarragon
- 1 tablespoon organic dill
- 1 tablespoon organic basil
- 2 tablespoons apple cider vinegar
- 2 tablespoons garlic-infused olive oil

Instructions:

- Switch on the oven, then set it to 350 degrees F, and let it preheat.
- Take a 10-by-12 inches roasting tray, arrange cherry tomatoes in it, add red bell pepper, top with chicken thighs, and then add fennel.
- Drizzle garlic oil and vinegar over chicken, season with salt, black pepper, and paprika, then toss all the ingredients until mixed and spread evenly.
- Roast the chicken thighs and vegetables for 1 hour, flipping the chicken and stirring the vegetables halfway through, and basting with cooking juices.
- Add green beans to the roasting pan when 5 minutes of the cooking time is left and baste them with cooking liquid.
- When done, garnish the chicken and vegetables with tarragon, dill, and basil, drizzle with some more garlic-infused oil and serve.

Grilled Sauerkraut Avocado Sandwich

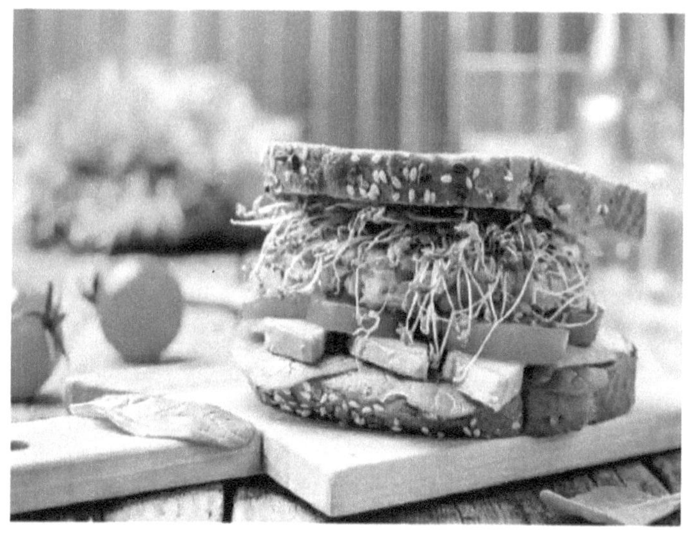

Serves: 4 sandwiches; Prep time: 10 minutes; Cooking time: 14 minutes; Total time: 24 minutes;

Nutritional values per serving:

Calories: 319 Cal; Fat: 14 g; Carbs: 39 g; Protein: 10 g; Fiber: 11 g;

Ingredients:

- 8 slices of pumpernickel bread
- 1 cup organic sauerkraut, drained
- 1 medium organic avocado, peeled, pitted and sliced
- 8 tablespoons unsalted butter
- 1 cup roasted garlic hummus

Instructions:

1. Switch on the oven, then set it to 450 degrees F, and then let it preheat.
2. Prepare the bread slices and for this, spread 1 tablespoon butter on one side of each slice, then place four slices of bread on a baking sheet, butter-side down, and spread half of the hummus on the slices on the baking sheet.
3. Drain the sauerkraut, rinse it lightly, squeeze out all the moisture, then distribute evenly over the hummus on each slice of bread and top with avocado slices.
4. Spread remaining hummus on the one side of the remaining slices of bread without butter side, place them over avocado slices, hummus side down, and bake for 14 minutes until crispy and brown, flipping the sandwiches halfway through.
5. Serve straight away.

6. ***Tempeh Hash with Brussels Sprouts***

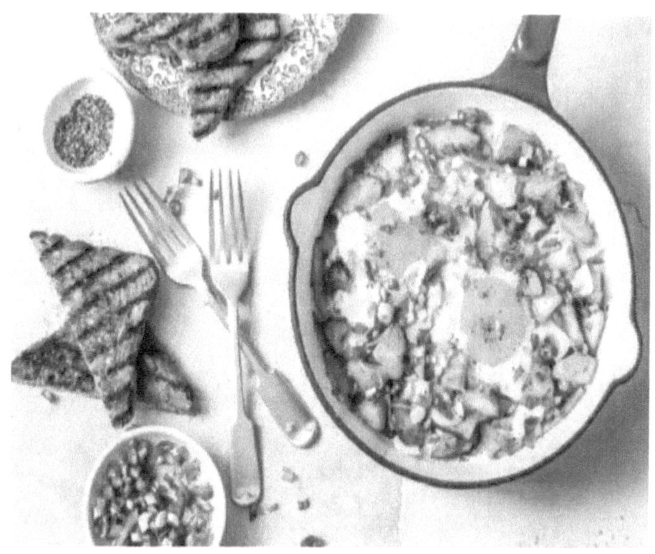

Serves: 4; Prep time: 10 minutes; Cooking time: 33 minutes; Total time: 43 minutes;

Nutritional values per serving:

Calories: 590 Cal; Fat: 29 g; Carbs: 75 g; Protein: 31 g; Fiber: 29 g;

Ingredients:

- 8 ounces tempeh, crumbled
- 1 cup diced organic shallot
- 2 cups shredded organic Brussels sprouts
- 3 cups diced organic potatoes, about 1-inch pieces

- 1/2 teaspoon garlic powder
- ½ teaspoon salt
- 1/3 teaspoon ground black pepper
- 2 teaspoons raw honey
- 1/2 teaspoon smoked paprika
- 1/2 teaspoon dried oregano
- 2 tablespoons tamari
- 1 tablespoon olive oil
- 1 tablespoon organic mustard

Instructions:

1. Place a large skillet pan over medium heat, add oil and when hot, add tempeh and cook it for 5 to 7 minutes until lightly brown.
2. Meanwhile, take a medium bowl, add mustard, honey, and tamari in it and then whisk in the garlic, paprika, and oregano until combined.
3. When the tempeh has cooked, transfer it to the bowl containing mustard mixture and toss until well coated, set aside until required.
4. Add potatoes into the pan, season with ¼ teaspoon salt and black pepper, stir well and cook for 10 to 15 minutes until potatoes are tender.
5. When potatoes have cooked, transfer them to a plate, set aside until required, then add shallots into the pan, season with remaining salt, and cook for 3 minutes until softened.
6. Add sprouts into the pan, stir until just mixed, and continue cooking for 5 minutes.
7. Return potatoes and tempeh into the pan, stir well, and cook for 2 minutes until thoroughly heated.

- Serve straight away.

Shrimp in Butter Sauce

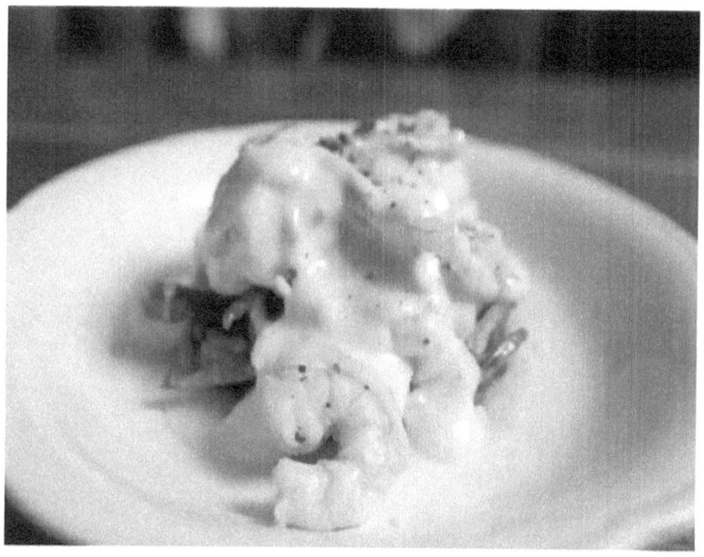

Serves: 4; Prep time: 5 minutes; Cooking time: 7 minutes; Total time: 12 minutes;

Nutritional values per serving:

Calories: 190 Cal; Fat: 13.3 g; Carbs: 1.8 g; Protein: 15.7 g; Fiber: 0.3 g;

Ingredients:

- 2 pounds wild-caught shrimp, peeled, deveined
- 1/2 cup chopped organic parsley
- 6 teaspoons minced organic garlic
- 1 ½ teaspoon salt
- 1 teaspoon ground black pepper

- 1 teaspoon red pepper flakes
- 4 tablespoons lemon juice
- 2 tablespoons olive oil
- 6 tablespoons unsalted butter, cut into cubes
- 2 tablespoons caper brine

Instructions:

1. Take a large skillet pan, place it over high heat, add oil and red pepper flakes and cook for 1 minute until fragrant.
2. Add shrimps, spread them evenly, and cook for 1 minute per side.
3. Add garlic, salt, and black pepper, drizzle with caper brine and lemon juice, stir well and cook for another minute.
4. Then add butter, half of the parsley, stir until mixed, swirl the pan to melt the butter, and it melts, add the remaining parsley and stir until combined.
5. Remove pan from heat and serve straight away.

Mushroom and Leek Soup

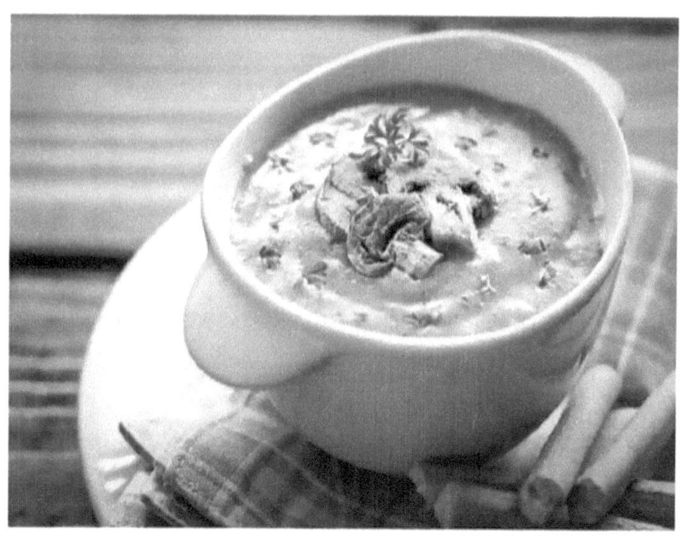

Serves: 4; Prep time: 10 minutes; Cooking time: 30 minutes; Total time: 40 minutes;

Nutritional values per serving:

Calories: 240 Cal; Fat: 10.1 g; Carbs: 25.6 g; Protein: 13.1 g; Fiber: 2.5 g;

Ingredients:

- 4 large organic portabello mushroom caps, destemmed, chopped
- 2 medium organic white onion , peeled, chopped
- 2 medium organic leek, chopped
- 3 teaspoons minced organic garlic

- 2 tablespoon chopped fresh organic parsley
- 2/3 teaspoon ground black pepper
- 2 teaspoon salt
- 4 sprigs of organic thyme
- 4 tablespoons heavy cream
- 6 cups of chicken bone broth

Instructions:

1. Take a stockpot, place it over medium heat, add oil and when hot, add onion, garlic, and leek and cook for 5 minutes until vegetables start to soften.
2. Add mushrooms, continue cooking for 4 minutes until mushrooms have started to brown, then add thyme sprig, pour in the stock, and simmer the soup for 15 to 20 minutes.
3. Then remove the pot from heat, take out and discard thyme sprigs from the soup and puree the soup by using an immersion blender until smooth.
4. Season the soup with salt and black pepper, add heavy cream, stir well until incorporated, and taste the soup to adjust seasoning.
5. Ladle soup into four bowls, garnish with parsley and serve.

Chicken Meatballs with Greens

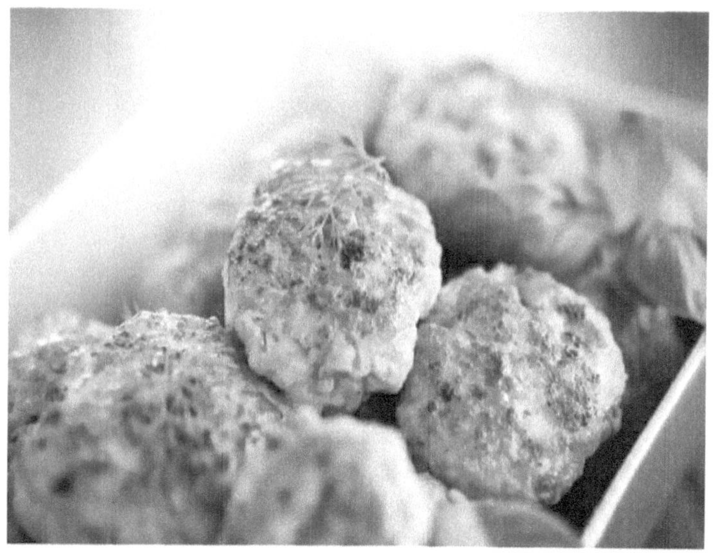

Serves: 4; Prep time: 10 minutes; Cooking time: 15 minutes; Total time: 25 minutes;

Nutritional values per serving:

Calories: 192 Cal; Fat: 8 g; Carbs: 3 g; Protein: 26 g; Fiber: 1 g;

Ingredients:

- 1 pound antibiotic-free, pasteurized ground chicken
- 2 heads of organic bok choy, leaves separated, halved lengthwise
- 4 organic spring onions, finely chopped
- 4 slices of organic ginger

- 1 teaspoon minced organic garlic
- 3/4-inch organic ginger root, peeled, grated
- 1 organic red chili, deseeded, chopped
- ¾ teaspoon salt
- ½ teaspoon ground black pepper
- 1 lime, juiced
- 2 tablespoons rapeseed oil
- 1 tablespoon soy sauce
- 5 cups of chicken bone broth

Instructions:

1. Prepare the meatballs and for this, place ground chicken in a bowl, add minced garlic, grated ginger, half of the spring onion and soy sauce, mix well and then shape the mixture into meatballs of walnut size.
2. Take a medium saucepan, place it over medium heat, add 1 tablespoon oil and when hot, add meatballs in a single layer and cook for 5 minutes until nicely golden brown on all sides.
3. When done, transfer chicken meatballs to a plate and cook remaining meatballs in the same manner by using remaining oil.
4. Then pour chicken stock into the pan, bring it to simmer, then add ginger slices and meatballs and cook for 3 minutes.
5. Add remaining spring onion, red chili, and bok choy and continue cooking for 5 minutes.
6. Stir in lime juice, season with salt and black pepper, and remove the pan from heat.
7. Serve chicken meatballs and greens with zucchini noodles.

Veggie Stir Fry

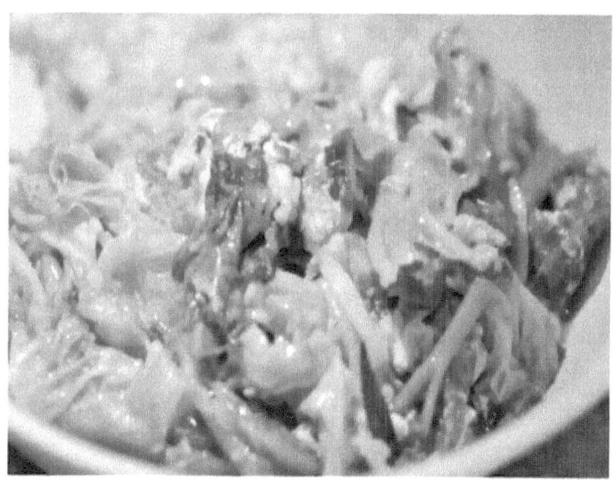

Serves: 4; Prep time: 5 minutes; Cooking time: 12 minutes; Total time: 17 minutes;

Nutritional values per serving:

Calories: 83 Cal; Fat: 0.5 g; Carbs: 16.3 g; Protein: 2.6 g; Fiber: 4.7 g;

Ingredients:

- 4 cups sliced organic cabbage
- 2 cups sliced organic white onion
- 2 cups diced organic celery
- 2 cups sliced organic mushrooms
- ½ teaspoon of sea salt
- ¼ teaspoon cracked black pepper
- 4 tablespoons water, divided

Instructions:

1. Take a skillet pan, place it over medium heat, let it heat for 1 minute, then add onion and cook for 3 to 4 minutes until onions are light brown and start to stick to the skillet.
2. Add 2 tablespoons water, stir well, continue cooking the onions, then add remaining water and continue cooking until onions are browned and start to stick, stirring frequently.
3. Then add cabbage, celery, and mushrooms, season with salt and black pepper, mix well and continue cooking for 5 minutes until vegetables have softened.
4. Serve straight away.

Roasted Broccoli

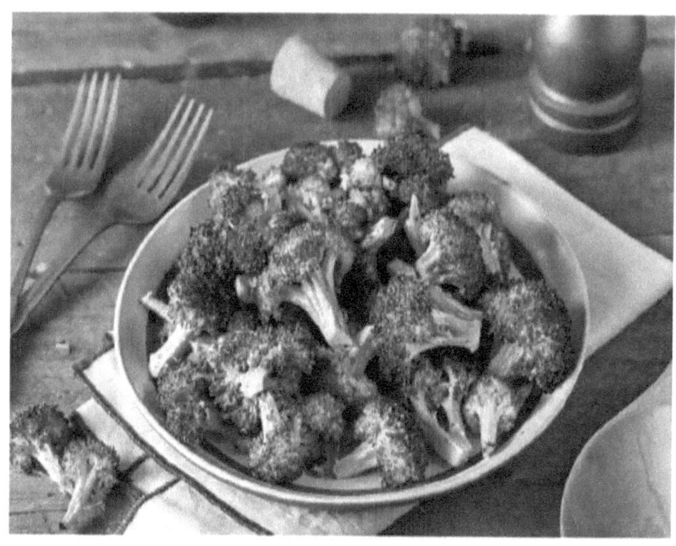

Serves: 4; Prep time: 10 minutes; Cooking time: 20 minutes; Total time: 30 minutes;

Nutritional values per serving:

Calories: 66 Cal; Fat: 3.8 g; Carbs: 7.3 g; Protein: 3 g; Fiber: 2.7 g;

Ingredients:

- 4 heads of organic broccoli, cut into florets
- 4 teaspoons minced organic garlic
- 1 ¼ teaspoon cracked black pepper
- 1 ¾ teaspoon salt
- ¼ teaspoon red pepper flakes

- 6 tablespoons melted coconut oil
- 2 teaspoons lemon juice

Instructions:

1. Switch on the oven, then set it to 400 degrees F, and let it preheat.
2. Meanwhile, place broccoli florets in a large bowl, season with salt, black pepper, and garlic, drizzle with oil and toss until well coated.
3. Take a large rimmed baking sheet, spread prepared broccoli florets on it in a single layer, and bake for 15 2o 20 minutes until fork-tender and edges of florets are lightly browned, turning the florets halfway through.
4. Sprinkle red pepper flakes over broccoli florets and serve.

5. ***Herb Crusted Salmon***

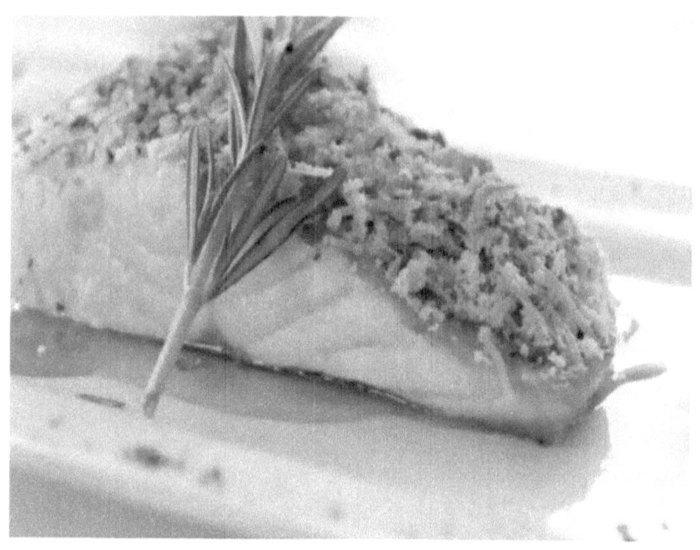

Serves: 4; Prep time: 10 minutes; Cooking time: 15 minutes; Total time: 25 minutes;

Nutritional values per serving:

Calories: 360.8 Cal; Fat: 26.1 g; Carbs: 6.3 g; Protein: 25.3 g; Fiber: 3 g;

Ingredients:

For the Salmon:

4 wild-caught salmon fillets, each about 6-ounces

4 tablespoons fresh parsley

2 tablespoons coconut flour

¾ teaspoon cracked black pepper

1 teaspoon salt

2 tablespoons olive oil

2 tablespoon organic mustard

    For the Salad:

½ of medium organic red onion, peeled, thinly sliced

4 cups organic arugula

2 organic lemons, juiced

¼ teaspoon cracked black pepper

½ teaspoon salt

2 tablespoons apple cider vinegar

2 tablespoons olive oil

Instructions:

- Switch on the oven, then set it to 450 degrees F and let it preheat.
- Meanwhile, take a baking sheet, line it with aluminum foil, place salmon fillets on it, drizzle oil and mustard on salmon and then rub into the meat.
- Place flour in a small bowl, add salt, black pepper, and parsley and stir until mixed.
- Spoon the coconut flour mixture evenly on each salmon fillet, press it into the salmon and then bake for 10 to 15 minutes until salmon has cooked to the desired level.
- Meanwhile, prepare the salmon and for this, place onion in a salad bowl, add arugula, sprinkle with black pepper and salt, drizzle with vinegar and oil and toss until well combined.
- Divide salad evenly between four plates, top with roasted salmon

and serve.

Dinner Recipes

Veggies and Shrimp with Rice Noodles

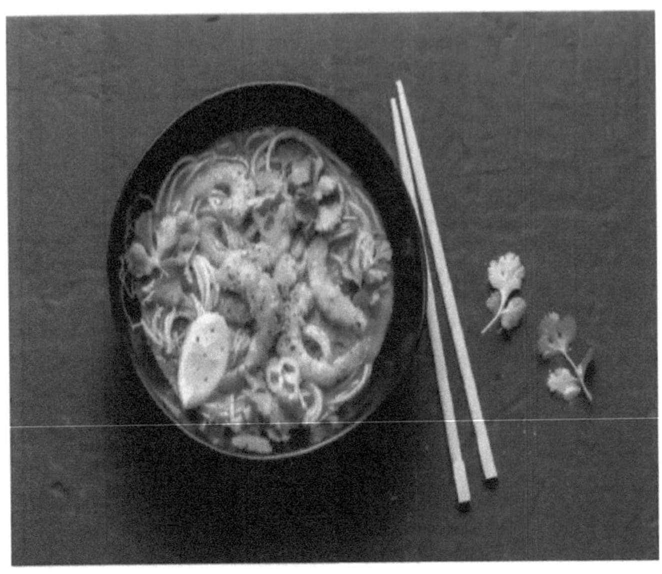

Serves: 4; Prep time: 10 minutes; Cooking time: 23 minutes; Total time: 33 minutes;

Nutritional values per serving:

Calories: 488 Cal; Fat: 14.1 g; Carbs: 60 g; Protein: 30.5 g; Fiber: 3.6 g;

Ingredients:

- 1 pound large wild-caught shrimp, peeled, deveined
- 1 cup of shredded organic carrots
- 2 small organic scallions, sliced

- 1 cup organic mushrooms, sliced
- 1 cup organic pea pods
- ¼ cup fresh organic basil, chopped
- ¼ teaspoon ground black pepper
- ½ teaspoon ground ginger
- 1 ½ teaspoons sea salt, divided
- 1 tablespoon sesame seeds
- 2 tablespoons coconut oil, divided
- 2 teaspoons molasses
- 1 tablespoon apple cider vinegar
- 1 tablespoon sesame oil
- 1 cup vegetable broth
- 8 ounces uncooked rice noodles

Instructions:

1. Place a medium pot half-full with water over medium heat, bring it to boil, then add rice noodles and remove the pot from heat.
2. Let the noodles sit in water for 5 minutes, then drain and rinse them in cold water and set aside until required.
3. Take a large skillet pan, place it over medium-high heat, add 1 tablespoon of coconut oil and let heat until it melts.
4. Season shrimps with black pepper and ½ teaspoon salt, add the shrimps to the skillet pan and cook for 10 minutes until pink and firm.
5. When done, transfer shrimps to a plate, switch the heat to medium level, add remaining oil in the pan, then add scallion, carrots, mushrooms, and pea pods and cook for 3 minutes until tender.
6. Meanwhile, prepare the sauce and for this, pour the broth in a bowl, add ginger, remaining salt, molasses, vinegar, and sesame oil and whisk until combined.
7. Pour the sauce evenly over the vegetables in the skillet, add rice noodles and shrimps, toss until well coated, and cook for 3

minutes until thoroughly heated.

8. Remove pan from heat, garnish shrimps and rice noodles with sesame seeds and basil and serve.

Chicken Thighs with Pineapple Salsa

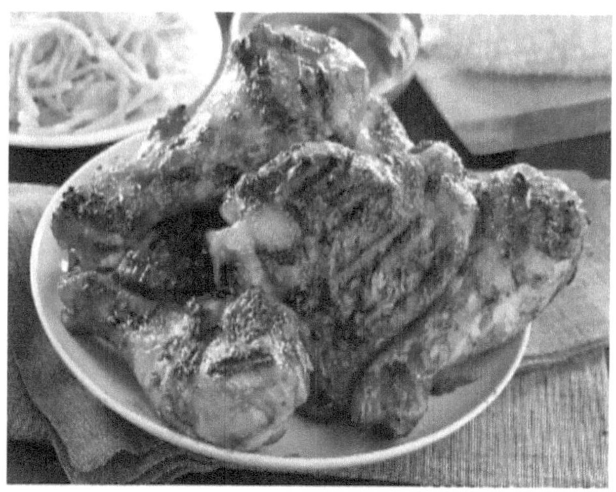

Serves: 4; Prep time: 10 minutes; Cooking time: 15 minutes; Total time: 25 minutes;

Nutritional values per serving:

Calories: 253 Cal; Fat: 13 g; Carbs: 8 g; Protein: 26 g; Fiber: 1 g;

Ingredients:

For the Chicken:

- 2 pounds antibiotic-free, pasteurized chicken thighs, bone-in, skin-on
- ½ teaspoon of sea salt
- ½ teaspoon garlic powder
- ½ teaspoon ginger powder

For the Salsa:

- 1 bunch of organic green onions, chopped
- 1 bunch of organic radishes, tops removed
- 1 organic avocado, pitted
- 1 medium organic cucumber
- ½ of a large organic pineapple
- 2 tablespoons chopped organic mint leaves
- ½ teaspoon of sea salt
- ½ teaspoon ginger powder
- ½ teaspoon minced garlic
- ½ of organic lemon, juiced

Instructions:

- Set the grill, brush the grilling rack generously with oil and let it preheat over medium heat.
- Meanwhile, place salt, garlic powder, and ginger powder in a shallow bowl and then stir well
- Coat the chicken thighs with the spice mixture, and rub it into the chicken.
- Place seasoned chicken thighs on the hot grilling rack, skin-side down, and cook for 5 to 7 minutes until the skin on chicken thighs start to get crisp.
- Then flip the chicken thighs and cook for another 5 to 7 minutes until a meat thermometer inserted into the thickest part of the thigh reads 165 degrees F.
- While chicken is grilling, prepare the salsa and for this, cut avocado, cucumber, radish, and pineapple into ½-inch chunks, place into a bowl, add remaining ingredients of salsa and stir until well combined.
- Serve grilled chicken thighs with prepared salsa.

Salmon with Green Beans

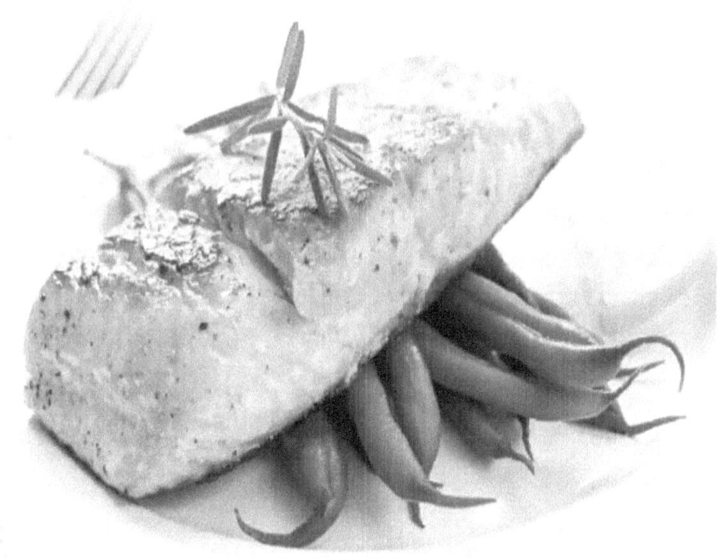

Serves: 4; Prep time: 10 minutes; Cooking time: 20 minutes; Total time: 30 minutes;

Nutritional values per serving:

Calories: 305 Cal; Fat: 18 g; Carbs: 6 g; Protein: 29 g; Fiber: 2 g;

Ingredients:

- 4 wild-caught salmon fillets
- 2 cups organic green beans, ends trimmed
- 1 teaspoon cracked black pepper
- 4 teaspoons dried tarragon

- 1 teaspoon sea salt, divided
- 1 teaspoon olive oil
- 4 wedges of lemon, for serving

Instructions:

1. Switch on the oven, then set it to 350 degrees F, and let it preheat.
2. Meanwhile, prepare salmon, and for this, season salmon with ½ teaspoon each of salt and black pepper and then sprinkle with 1 teaspoon of dried tarragon per fillet.
3. Take a baking sheet, line it with aluminum foil, place prepared salmon fillets on it and bake for 20 minutes until cooked.
4. Meanwhile, prepare green beans and for this, place a pot half-full with water over medium-high heat, bring it to boil, then add green beans and boil for 3 minutes until vibrant.
5. Drain the green beans, transfer them to a bowl, season with remaining salt, and drizzle with oil and toss until mixed.
6. Divide green beans evenly between four plates, add roasted salmon and serve with a lemon wedge.

Chicken Piccata

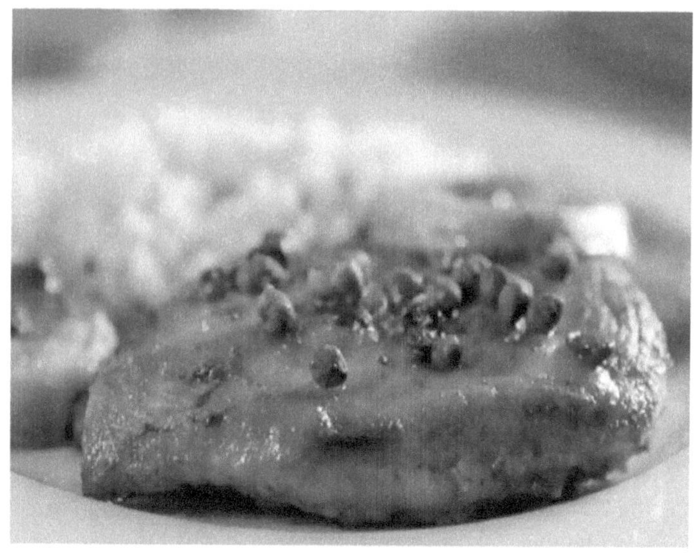

Serves: 4; Prep time: 10 minutes; Cooking time: 18 minutes; Total time: 28 minutes;

Nutritional values per serving:

Calories: 520 Cal; Fat: 12.3 g; Carbs: 47.8 g; Protein: 47.1 g; Fiber: 3 g;

Ingredients:

- 1 pound antibiotic-free, pasteurized chicken tenderloins, boneless, skinless
- 2 medium organic shallots, peeled, chopped
- 2 tablespoons capers
- ¼ teaspoon cracked black pepper

- ½ teaspoon salt
- ⅓ cup brown rice flour
- 3 tablespoons lemon juice
- ¼ cup of coconut oil
- ¾ cup of chicken bone broth

Instructions:

- Prepare chicken thighs, and for this, wrap each chicken thigh in a plastic wrap and pound with a meat mallet until ¼-inch thick.
- Place rice flour in a shallow bowl, then add salt and black pepper and stir until mixed.
- Take a large skillet pan, place it over medium heat, add coconut oil, and let it heat until melts.
- Coat chicken thighs evenly into the rice flour mixture, add to the hot skillet pan in a single layer, then switch heat to medium-high level and cook for 5 minutes per side until chicken is golden brown.
- When done, transfer chicken thighs to a plate and cook the remaining chicken thighs in the same manner.
- Then add shallots into the pan, cook for 2 minutes until sautéed, then return chicken thighs in it, add capers, drizzle with lemon juice, pour in the broth, and stir well.
- Simmer the chicken for 5 minutes or until cooking sauce is slightly thick.
- Serve straight away.

Creamy Potato and Chicken Soup

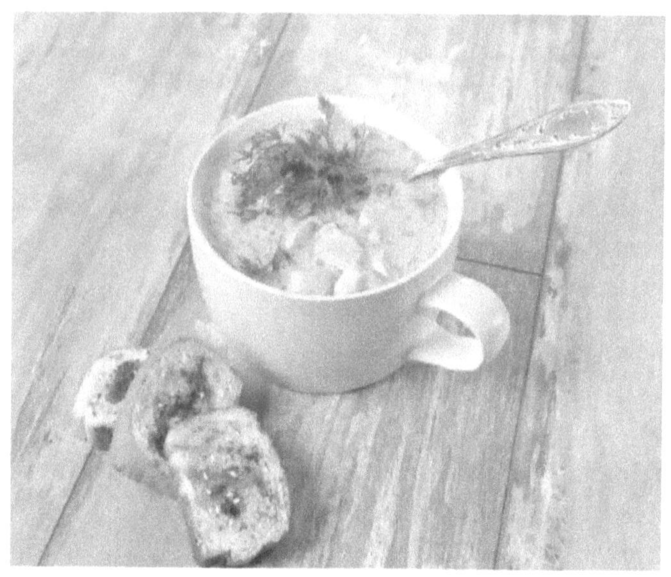

Serves: 4; Prep time: 10 minutes; Cooking time: 30 minutes; Total time: 40 minutes;

Nutritional values per serving:

Calories: 732.2 Cal; Fat: 23.6 g; Carbs: 66 g; Protein: 64.1 g; Fiber: 12.4 g;

Ingredients:

- 6 ounces nitrate-free, pasteurized bacon, diced
- 3 cups cooked antibiotic-free, pasteurized chicken, shredded
- 1 medium organic white onion, peeled, chopped
- 2 tablespoons sliced organic green onions

- 3 cups white organic sweet potatoes, peeled, cubed
- 1 medium organic carrot, peeled, chopped
- 3 cups organic parsnips, peeled, cubed
- 1 ½ stalk of organic celery, chopped
- 1 teaspoon minced organic garlic
- 1/3 teaspoon cracked black pepper
- 2/3 teaspoon salt
- 1 bay leaf
- 1 organic lemon, juiced
- 4 cups of chicken bone broth

Instructions:

1. Take a medium pot, place it over medium heat and when hot, add bacon, then cook for 5 minutes until crispy and transfer bacon to a plate lined with paper towels, set aside until required.
2. Add celery, onion, and carrot into the pot, stir well and cook for 5 to 7 minutes until vegetables have softened.
3. Add garlic into the pot, cook it for 1 minute until fragrant, then switch heat to medium-high level, add potatoes, parsnip and bay leaves, pour in the broth, stir well and bring the mixture to boil.
4. Lower heat to medium level and simmer vegetables for 10 minutes until tender.
5. Remove pot from the heat, discard bay leaf from the soup, and use an immersion blender to puree the soup until smooth.
6. Season soup with salt and black pepper, stir in lemon juice, then add chicken and stir until mixed.
7. Return pot over medium heat, cook the soup for 5 minutes until thoroughly warm.
8. Ladle soup into bowls, top with cooked bacon and green onion and serve.

Superfood Burger

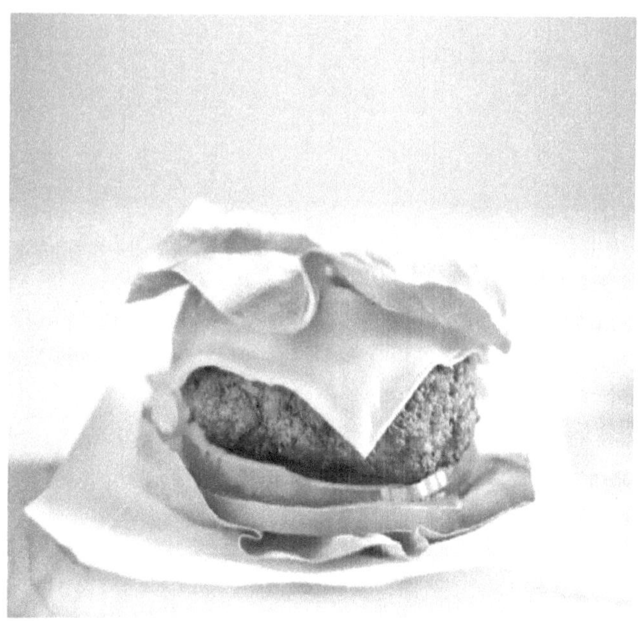

Serves: 4 burgers; Prep time: 10 minutes; Cooking time: 10 minutes; Total time: 20 minutes;

Nutritional values per serving:

Calories: 364.3 Cal; Fat: 22 g; Carbs: 6.4 g; Protein: 35.5 g; Fiber: 3.2 g;

Ingredients:

- 1¼ pounds grass-fed ground beef
- ½ cup organic sauerkraut, drained
- ½ a medium organic white onion , peeled, sliced

- ½ cup organic watercress
- ½ of head organic romaine lettuce
- 2/3 teaspoon salt
- ¼ cup of organic mustard

Instructions:

1. Set the grill, brush its grilling rack generously with oil and let preheat over medium-high heat setting.
2. Then shape the beef into four patties, place them on the grilling rack and cook them for 5 minutes per side until browned and thoroughly cooked.
3. Divide lettuce leaves into four sections as they will serve as a burger bun, then place a patty on it, top with onion, watercress, and sauerkraut and serve.

Taco Soup

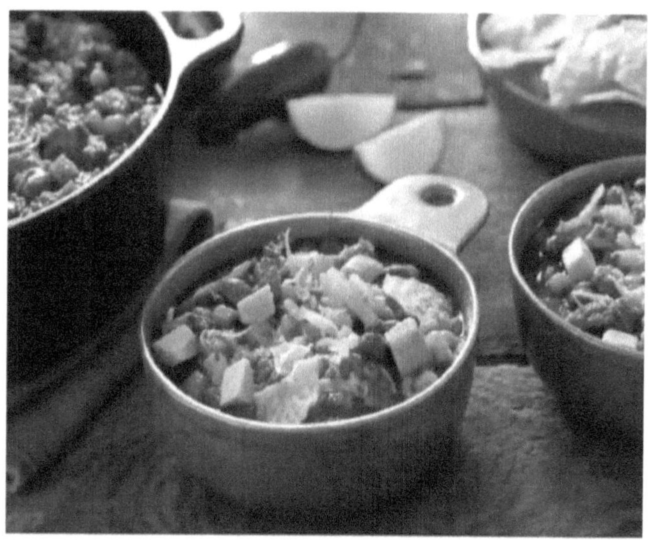

Serves: 4; Prep time: 10 minutes; Cooking time: 25 minutes; Total time: 35 minutes;

Nutritional values per serving:

Calories: 510.5 Cal; Fat: 32 g; Carbs: 18 g; Protein: 38.3 g; Fiber: 8.8 g;

Ingredients:

- 1 pound grass-fed ground beef
- 2 organic avocados, pitted, chopped
- 2 organic zucchini, chopped into quarter moons
- 1 bunch of organic scallions, chopped
- 4 organic radishes, ¼-inch thinly sliced

- 2 large organic carrots, cut into ¼-inch thick matchsticks
- 1 bunch of organic cilantro, chopped
- 1 teaspoon of sea salt
- 2 teaspoons ground cumin
- 2 organic limes, halved
- 4 cups of chicken bone broth

Instructions:

1. Take a large saucepan, place it over medium-high heat, add zucchini, pour in the broth, and bring the mixture to boil.
2. Then switch heat to medium-low level and simmer the mixture for 10 minutes, covering the saucepan.
3. Meanwhile, place a skillet pan over medium heat, grease with oil and when hot, add white parts of scallions and beef, stir well and cook for 7 to 10 minutes until beef has thoroughly cooked.
4. Then add beef into the saucepan, season with salt and cumin, add radish and carrot, stir well and remove the pan from heat.
5. Ladle soup into four bowls, top with green parts of scallions, cilantro and avocado and serve with lime.

Thai Chickpea Curry

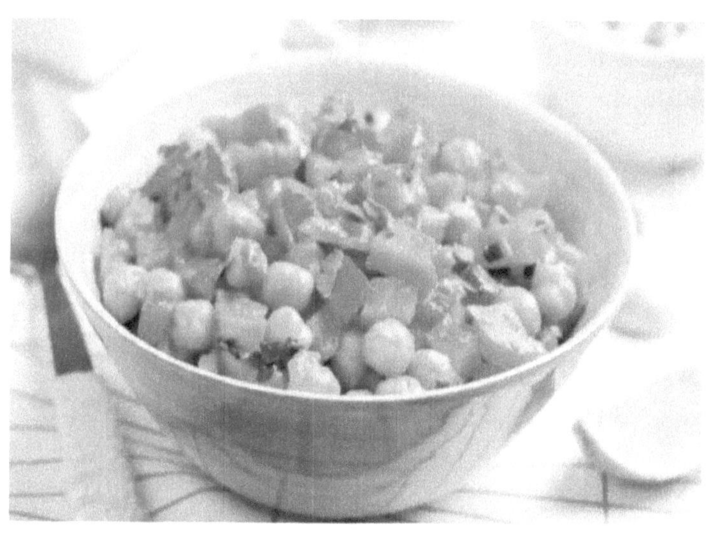

Serves: 4; Prep time: 10 minutes; Cooking time: 26 minutes; Total time: 36 minutes;

Nutritional values per serving:

Calories: 389 Cal; Fat: 12.7 g; Carbs: 42.1 g; Protein: 12.2 g; Fiber: 11.5 g;

Ingredients:

- 15 ounces cooked chickpeas
- 3/4 cup diced organic green onion and more for topping
- 1 cup of frozen organic peas
- 1 cup diced organic carrots
- 1 medium organic red bell pepper, cored, sliced
- 1 tablespoon minced organic ginger

- 1 ½ teaspoon minced organic garlic
- 1/2 teaspoon salt
- 2 tablespoons green curry paste
- 3 tablespoons diced fresh organic basil
- 1/2 tablespoon ground turmeric
- 1 lime, juiced
- 1 tablespoon soy sauce
- 2 stalks of organic lemongrass, minced
- 2 teaspoons coconut oil
- 15 ounces coconut milk, unsweetened
- 1/2 cup vegetarian broth
- 4 teaspoons hot sauce

Instructions:

1. Take a large pot, place it over medium-high heat, add oil and when hot, add onion, garlic, ginger, carrot, lemongrass, basil, and cook for 5 minutes until onions are slightly brown.
2. Stir in turmeric and green curry paste, cook for 30 seconds until fragrant, then add remaining ingredients, except for peas and hot sauce, stir well and bring the mixture to boil.
3. Switch heat to medium-low level and simmer the soup for 20 minutes until carrots are tender, uncovering the pot.
4. Then stir in peas and remove the pot from heat.
5. Ladle the curry into bowls, top with green onions, drizzle with hot sauce and serve with fried cauliflower rice.

Turkey Soup

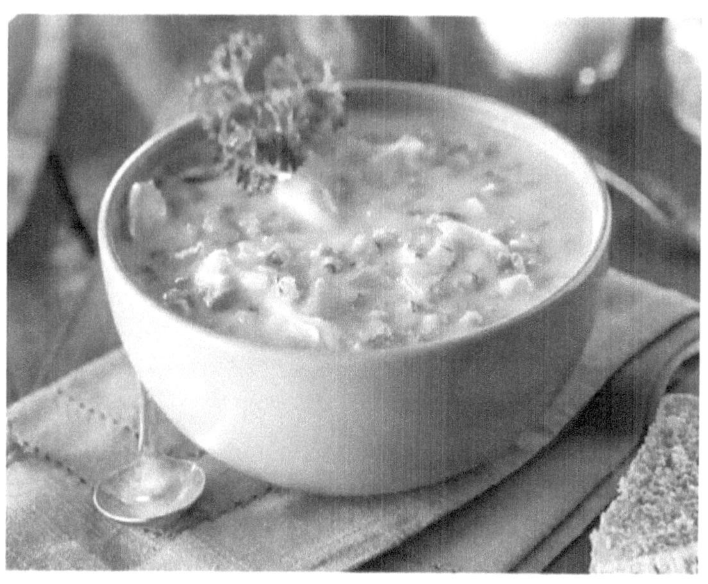

Serves: 4; Prep time: 5 minutes; Cooking time: 15 minutes; Total time: 20 minutes;

Nutritional values per serving:

Calories: 170 Cal; Fat: 6.2 g; Carbs: 8.9 g; Protein: 19.6 g; Fiber: 2 g;

Ingredients:

- 1 cup cooked, shredded, pasteurized turkey meat
- 1/3 cup organic shiitake mushrooms, halved
- 1/3 cup organic cherry tomatoes
- 2 handfuls of organic sprouts

- 1 medium organic white onion , peeled, sliced
- 1 medium organic green bell pepper
- 1 ½ teaspoon minced organic garlic
- 1-inch piece of organic ginger, julienned
- ½ teaspoon salt
- 1 1/2 tablespoons Thai green curry paste
- 1 teaspoon coconut oil
- 1 tablespoon soy sauce
- 4 cups of chicken bone broth
- 1/2 cup coconut milk, unsweetened
- ¼ cup organic cilantro

Instructions:

1. Take a large pot, place it over medium-high heat, add oil and when hot, add onion and cook for 5 minutes until onions begin to soften.
2. Add mushroom, continue cooking 5 minutes until softened, then add tomatoes, ginger, and garlic, and cook for 1 minute until fragrant.
3. Add turkey meat, salt, soy sauce, and curry paste, pour in the milk and chicken broth, and bring the soup to boil.
4. Reduce heat to medium-low level, simmer the soup for 2 minutes, then remove the pot from heat, add sprouts and bell pepper and stir well.
5. Taste the soup to adjust seasoning, then ladle soup into four bowls, top with cilantro and serve.

Coconut Chicken Curry

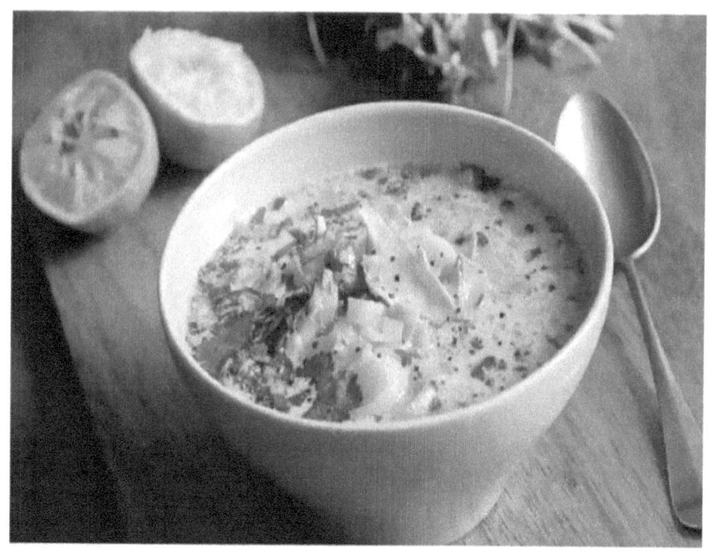

Serves: 4; Prep time: 10 minutes; Cooking time: 18 minutes; Total time: 28 minutes;

Nutritional values per serving:

Calories: 214 Cal; Fat: 11.7 g; Carbs: 14.4 g; Protein: 12.8 g; Fiber: 4.6 g;

Ingredients:

- 1 antibiotic-free, pasteurized chicken breast, cooked, diced
- 1 medium organic sweet potato, peeled, ½-inch cubed
- 1 medium organic avocado, peeled, sliced
- 2 medium stalks of organic celery, chopped
- 1/2 cup organic green onions, chopped

- 1 medium organic white onion , peeled, diced
- 1 teaspoon minced organic garlic
- 1/2 teaspoon onion powder
- 1/2 tablespoon cumin
- 1 teaspoon salt
- 1 tablespoon coriander
- 1/2 tablespoon ground turmeric
- 1 tablespoon coconut oil
- 1 cup of water
- 13.5 ounces coconut milk, unsweetened

Instructions:

1. Take a large skillet pan, place it over medium-high heat, add oil and when it melts, add garlic and cook for 1 minute until golden brown.
2. Add onion and continue cooking for 5 minutes until translucent, covering the pan.
3. Stir in onion powder, coriander, turmeric, and cumin, then add green onion, celery, and sweet potatoes, stir well until coated, then season with salt and pour in water.
4. Bring the mixture to boil, then switch heat to medium-low level and simmer the curry for 5 to 7 minutes until potatoes are tender.
5. Add chicken into the pan, pour in coconut milk, stir well and simmer for 3 minutes.
6. Remove pan from heat, top curry with avocado, and serve.

Veggie Packed Soup

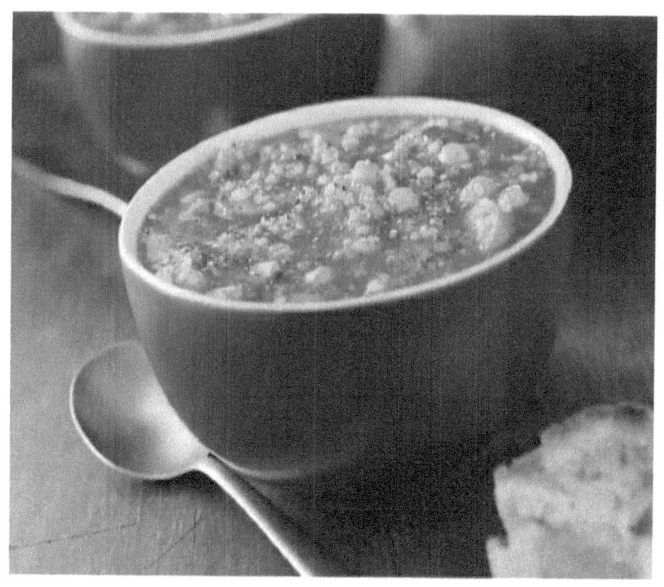

Serves: 4; Prep time: 10 minutes; Cooking time: 55 minutes; Total time: 1 hour and 5 minutes;

Nutritional values per serving:

Calories: 190 Cal; Fat: 4.6 g; Carbs: 30.6 g; Protein: 6.1 g; Fiber: 12 g;

Ingredients:

- 6 medium-large organic carrots, peeled, sliced
- 6 cups organic collard greens, stem removed
- 15 ounces diced organic tomatoes
- ½ teaspoon ground black pepper

- 1 teaspoon salt
- 1 1/2 teaspoon red chili powder
- 3 teaspoons smoked paprika
- 2 teaspoons cumin
- 1 cup uncooked quinoa
- 1 tablespoon pure maple syrup
- 3 tablespoons soy sauce
- 6 ounces tomato paste
- 3 tablespoons lemon juice
- 1 tablespoon coconut oil
- 10 ¼ cups water

Instructions:

1. Take a large pot, place it over medium heat, add oil and when it melts, add red chili powder, paprika, and cumin and cook for 30 seconds until fragrant.
2. Add carrots, pour in ¼ cup water, stir well and cook for 10 minutes, covering the pot.
3. Then switch heat to medium-high level, add remaining ingredients, stir well, and boil the soup for 8 minutes.
4. Switch heat to medium level and simmer the soup for 30 to 35 minutes until vegetables and quinoa are cooked, uncovering the pot.
5. Ladle soup into four bowls and serve.

Beef Ragu with Spaghetti Squash

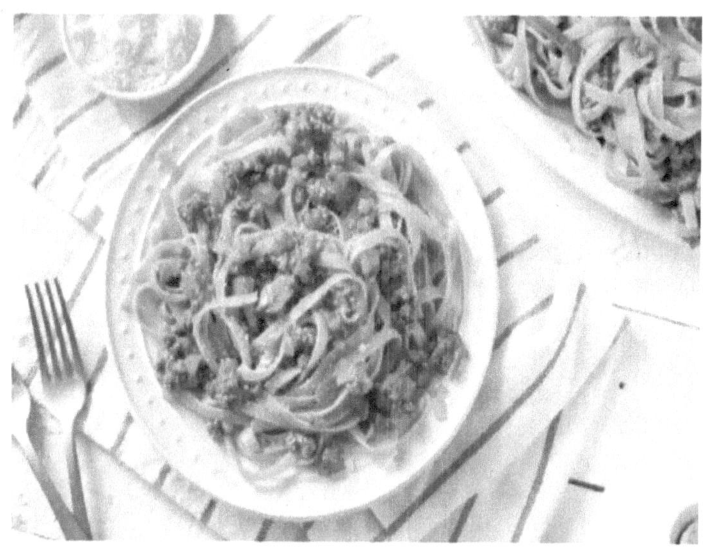

Serves: 4; Prep time: 10 minutes; Cooking time: 30 minutes; Total time: 40 minutes;

Nutritional values per serving:

Calories: 373 Cal; Fat: 22 g; Carbs: 17 g; Protein: 27 g; Fiber: 4 g;

Ingredients:

- 1 pound grass-fed ground beef
- 1 medium organic spaghetti squash
- 1 organic leek, chopped
- 2 sprigs sage leaves, minced
- 3 cups diced organic tomatoes

- 2 sprigs rosemary leaves, minced
- 1/3 teaspoon cracked black pepper
- 2 sprigs oregano leaves, minced
- 1 teaspoon salt
- 2 sprigs parsley leaves, minced
- 2 tablespoons coconut oil
- 2 teaspoons olive oil
- 1 teaspoon raw apple cider vinegar
- ½ cup beef bone broth
- 2 tablespoons grated parmesan cheese

Instructions:

1. Switch on the oven, turn it to broiling mode and let it preheat.
2. Place spaghetti squash on a baking tray, then place it under the broiler and roast for 30 minutes, turning halfway through.
3. Meanwhile, prepare the sauce and for this, take a large saucepan, place it medium heat, add coconut oil and when it melts, add beef and cook for 7 to 10 minutes until browned.
4. Transfer the cooked beef to a plate, set aside until required, then add olive oil into the pan along with leeks, and cook for 3 minutes until tender.
5. Then switch heat to medium-low level, return beef into the pan, add half of the sage, rosemary, oregano, and parsley, add tomatoes, pour in the broth, stir well and simmer for 10 minutes.
6. Season beef with ¾ teaspoon salt and black pepper, stir in vinegar, and remove the pan from heat.
7. When done, remove spaghetti sauce from the oven, carefully cut in half lengthwise, let it cool for 10 minutes until easily handle and then remove the seeds.
8. Season squash halves with remaining salt, then run fork to make noodles and evenly divide the noodles between four bowls.
9. Top with 1 cup of beef sauce, garnish with remaining sage, rosemary, oregano, and parsley, sprinkle with cheese and serve.

Almond-Crusted Cod with Greens

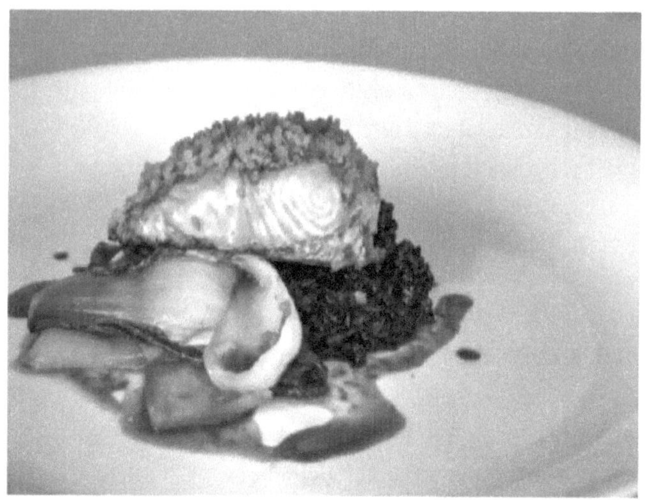

Serves: 4; Prep time: 10 minutes; Cooking time: 10 minutes; Total time: 20 minutes;

Nutritional values per serving:

Calories: 380 Cal; Fat: 22 g; Carbs: 14 g; Protein: 31 g; Fiber: 6 g;

Ingredients:

- 6 organic baby Bok choy, chopped, stems and leaves separated
- 2 medium organic red bell peppers, cored, sliced
- 1 1/4 pounds wild-caught cod fillets
- 2 sprigs rosemary leaves, minced
- 1/4 cup ground mustard
- 2 sprigs parsley leaves, minced

- 1 ¼ teaspoon sea salt
- 2 sprigs oregano leaves, minced
- ¼ teaspoon ground black pepper
- 1/2 cup slivered almonds, chopped
- 2 tablespoons apple cider vinegar
- 1 organic lemon, sliced into wedges
- 4 tablespoons avocado oil

Instructions:

1. Switch on the oven, then set it to 350 degrees F and let it preheat.
2. Place half of the rosemary, parsley, and oregano in a small bowl, add vinegar, mustard, black pepper, ¼ teaspoon salt and stir until well combined.
3. Take a 9 by 13 inches baking pan, grease it with 1 tablespoon oil, then place fillets it and top evenly with mustard mixture.
4. Sprinkle almonds on top of fillets, drizzle with 1 tablespoon oil, and season with ½ teaspoon salt and bake for 10 minutes until cooked.
5. Then switch on the broil and continue baking the fish for 2 minutes until the top is golden brown.
6. While fillets are baking, prepare vegetables and for this, take a large frying pan, place it over medium-high heat, add remaining oil and when hot, add bok choy stem and pepper and cook for 2 minutes until softened.
7. Then add bok choy leaves and continue cooking for 1 minute until its leaves wilts, then remove the pan from heat and season with remaining salt and black pepper.
8. Divide bok choy mixture evenly between four bowls, top with baked fillets, drizzle with juices, then garnish with remaining herbs and serve with a lemon wedge.

Desserts

Banana and Mint Chip Ice Cream

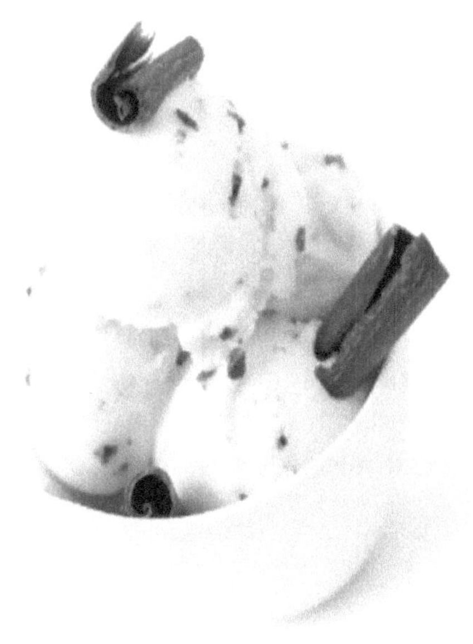

Serves: 4; Prep time: 6 hours and 5 minutes; Cooking time: 0 minutes; Total time: 6 hours and 5 minutes;

Nutritional values per serving:

Calories: 187 Cal; Fat: 7 g; Carbs: 31 g; Protein: 2 g; Fiber: 6 g;

Ingredients:

- 3 tablespoons chocolate chips, unsweetened
- 1 medium organic avocado
- 4 frozen organic bananas, peeled, cut into chunks
- 1/4 teaspoon matcha
- 1/2 teaspoon mint extract, unsweetened

Instructions:

1. Place all the ingredients for ice cream in a blender and pulse at high speed until creamy and smooth, scraping the sides as needed.
2. Take a freezer-safe container, transfer the ice cream mixture into it and freeze for a minimum of 6 hours or overnight.
3. When ready to eat, let the ice cream sit at room temperature for 10 minutes, then scoop it into bowls and serve.

Baked Stuffed Apples

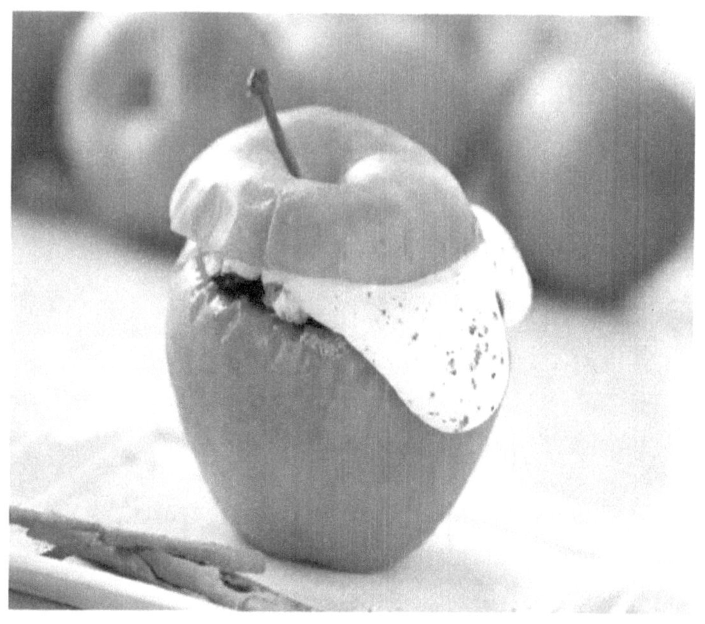

Serves: 4; Prep time: 10 minutes; Cooking time: 40 minutes; Total time: 50 minutes;

Nutritional values per serving:

Calories: 369 Cal; Fat: 12 g; Carbs: 59 g; Protein: 6.4 g; Fiber: 8.7 g;

Ingredients:

- 1 cups cooked steel-cut oatmeal, warm
- 4 organic gala apples
- 1 organic lemon, halved

- 1 ½ teaspoon grated orange zest
- 1/16 teaspoon ground black pepper
- ⅛ teaspoon ground cinnamon
- 1/16 teaspoon salt
- 4 tablespoons erythritol sweetener
- 3 tablespoons unsalted butter
- ¾ cup apple cider, unsweetened
- ¾ cup almond milk, heated
- Greek yogurt for serving

Instructions:

1. Switch on the oven, then set it to 375 degrees F, and let it preheat.
2. Prepare apples and for this, slice the bottom to make apples stand, then cut off the top third and make a 2-inch diameter cavity from the top by carving out the apple.
3. Remove seeds from carve-out apples, then dice it and set aside until required.
4. Take a small saucepan, place it over medium heat, add butter and when it melts, add 3 tablespoons sweetener, black pepper, and cinnamon, stir well and cook until smooth.
5. Remove the pan from heat and brush this butter mixture in the inside of the apples.
6. Take a baking dish, pour in apple cider, place apples in it, then cover with aluminum foil and bake for 30 minutes until apples are tender.
7. Meanwhile, take a small saucepan, place it over medium heat, pour in the milk and when hot, stir in reserve apples, remaining sweetener and orange rest and cook for 5 minutes, set aside until required.
8. Then uncover the baking dish, continue baking for 5 minutes, and when done, transfer apples to a plate.
9. Strain the cooking liquid into a small saucepan, place the pan over medium-low heat, bring it to boil, and continue cooking

for 5 minutes until thickened.

10. Assemble the apples and for this, stuff the apples evenly with oatmeal, then top with a dollop of yogurt, drizzle with orange zest-apple mixture and serve.

Poached Pears

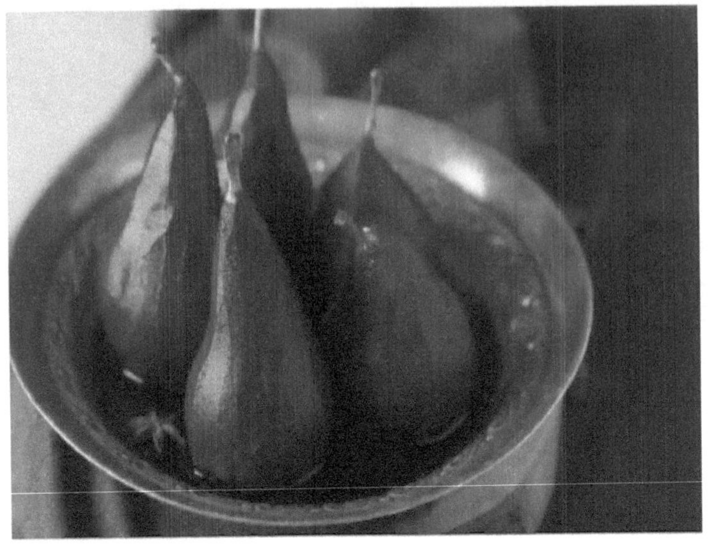

Serves: 4; Prep time: 10 minutes; Cooking time: 30 minutes; Total time: 40 minutes;

Nutritional values per serving:

Calories: 192 Cal; Fat: 0 g; Carbs: 46 g; Protein: 0 g; Fiber: 3.2 g;

Ingredients:

- 4 small organic pears, peeled, stalks left on
- 1 ½ tablespoon dried hibiscus flowers
- 4 ounces of coconut sugar
- 1 organic lemon, juiced, zested
- 2 ½ cup water

Instructions:

1. Take a small saucepan, place it over medium-high heat, pour in water, add sugar, lemon zest and hibiscus flower and bring the mixture to boil.
2. Then switch heat to medium-low level and simmer for 10 minutes until the sugar has dissolved and the liquid turned into deep red color.
3. Strain the liquid into a large pot, add lemon juice, stir well, then place the pan over medium heat, add pears in it in a single layer and simmer for 10 minutes until pears are fork-tender, covering the pot.
4. When done, transfer pears to a serving dish, then boil the cooking liquid until ¾ cup is left and let it cool.
5. Drizzle cooking liquid over pears and serve.

- ***Strawberries and Cream Muesli***

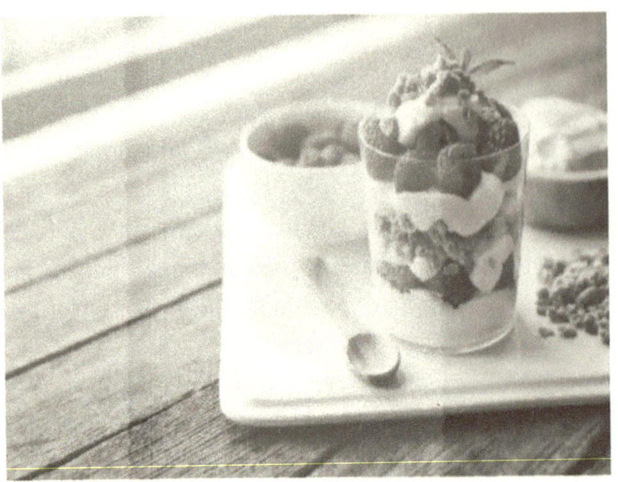

Serves: 4; Prep time: 5 hours and 10 minutes; Cooking time: 0 minutes; Total time: 5 hours and 10 minutes;

Nutritional values per serving:

Calories: 899 Cal; Fat: 57 g; Carbs: 83.2 g; Protein: 13.5 g; Fiber: 16.4 g;

Ingredients:

- 2 cups diced organic apples
- 2 cups old-fashioned oats
- 2 cups diced organic strawberries
- 2 tablespoons flax seeds
- ½ cup of coconut sugar
- 1/8 teaspoon salt

- 2 tablespoons chia seeds
- 2 cups shredded coconut, unsweetened
- 2 tablespoons vanilla extract, unsweetened
- 1 ½ cup almond milk, unsweetened
- 1 cup and 4 tablespoons heavy cream
- ½ cup coconut milk, unsweetened

Instructions:

1. Take four pint-jars and layer them with oats evenly, top with flaxseed and chia seeds, then add a layer of shredded coconut and top with apples and strawberries.
2. Take a pitcher, pour in remaining ingredients, mix well until sugar has dissolved, and then evenly pour over fruits and seeds in the pint-jars.
3. Cover the jars with lids, shake them until combined and refrigerate for a minimum of 5 hours or overnight.
4. Serve straight away.

Mango and Lime Sorbet

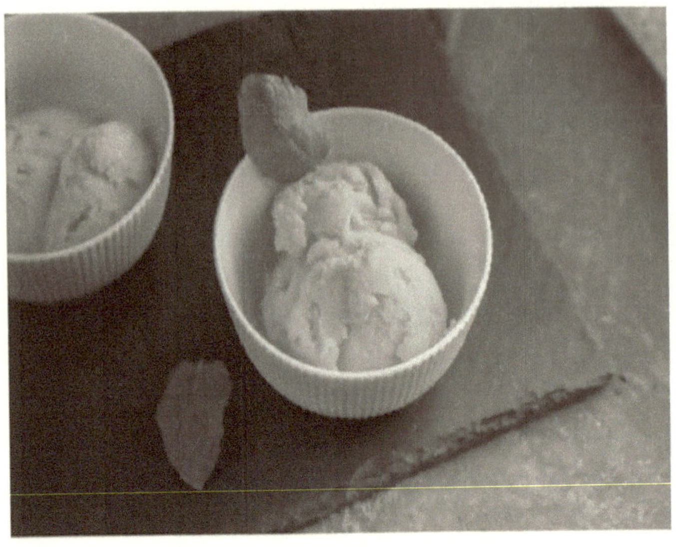

Serves: 4; Prep time: 40 minutes; Cooking time: 0 minutes; Total time: 40 minutes;

Nutritional values per serving:

Calories: 196 Cal; Fat: 9.4 g; Carbs: 27.3 g; Protein: 2.4 g; Fiber: 6.3 g;

Ingredients:

- 14 ounces fresh organic raspberries, and more for serving
- 2.2 pound frozen organic mango chunks
- 8 ounces grated coconut
- 2 tablespoons erythritol sweetener
- 2 limes, juiced, zested

- 1 cup of coconut water
- 4 tablespoons mint for garnishing

Instructions:

1. Place mango chunk in the freeze and let them chill for 20 minutes.
2. Add half of the mango chunks in a blender or food processor, add lime juice and lime zest, pulse until combined, and then gradually blend in coconut water until sorbet comes together.
3. Taste to adjust sweetener, then gradually blend in remaining mango chunks and coconut water until sorbet reached to desire consistency.
4. Evenly divide sorbet between four serving glasses, top with more raspberries, sprinkle with grated coconut and mint, and freeze for 10 minutes.
5. Serve immediately.

Salads

Sauerkraut Salad

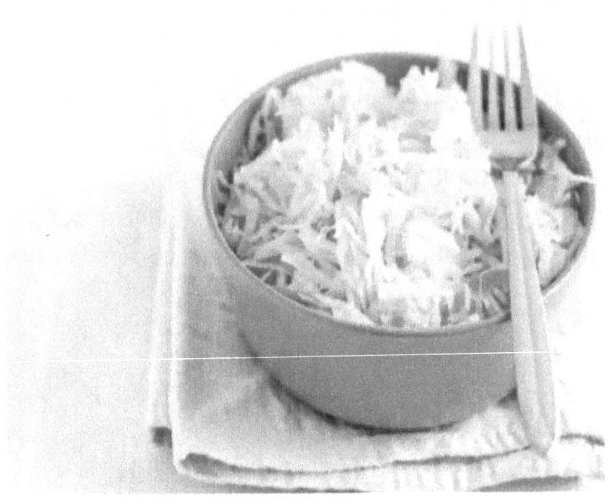

Serves: 4; Prep time: 10 minutes; Cooking time: 0 minutes; Total time: 10 minutes;

Nutritional values per serving:

Calories: 143 Cal; Fat: 0.6 g; Carbs: 32 g; Protein: 1.8 g; Fiber: 9.8 g;

Ingredients:

- 4 medium organic apples, cored, peel on, grated
- 2 medium organic carrots, peeled, grated
- 20-ounces organic sauerkraut

- 1 teaspoon minced organic garlic
- 1 cup chopped organic parsley

Instructions:

- Squeeze out liquid from sauerkraut as much as possible, then chop it finely and add to a bowl.
- Add remaining ingredients, toss until well mixed and taste to adjust seasoning with raw honey.
- Serve straight away or store in the refrigerator for two days.

Avocado and Papaya Salad

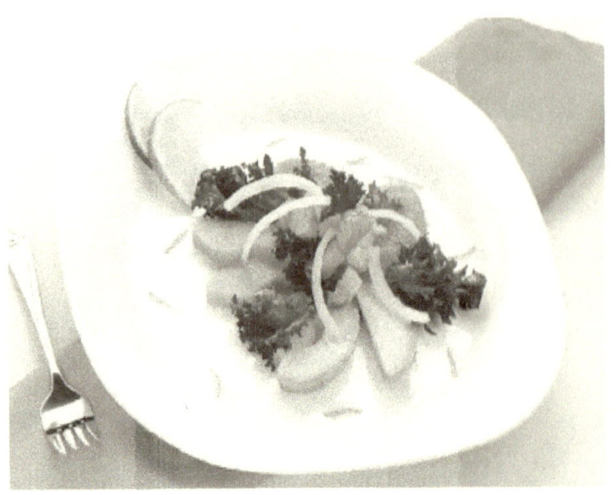

Serves: 4; Prep time: 10 minutes; Cooking time: 0 minutes; Total time: 10 minutes;

Nutritional values per serving:

Calories: 260 Cal; Fat: 22 g; Carbs: 11 g; Protein: 4 g; Fiber: 5 g;

Ingredients:

- 2 organic papayas, peeled, cored, thinly sliced lengthwise
- 2 organic avocados, peeled, pitted, thinly sliced lengthwise
- 4 ounces organic watercress, rinsed and chopped
- ½ cup organic mint leaves, chopped
- 4 tablespoons pumpkin seeds, toasted
- 1/3 teaspoon salt
- ¼ teaspoon ground black pepper

- 1 lime, juiced
- 2 tablespoons olive oil

Instructions:

1. Prepare the dressing and for this, place mint in a bowl, reserving 2 tablespoons for later use, then add lime juice and olive oil, season with black pepper, and stir until well combined.
2. Prepare the salad and for this, take a large salad bowl and add sliced papaya and avocado along with watercress, then add pumpkin seeds, drizzle with prepared salad dressing and toss until well combined.
3. Taste the salad to adjust seasoning and serve immediately.

Mango and Red Cabbage Salad

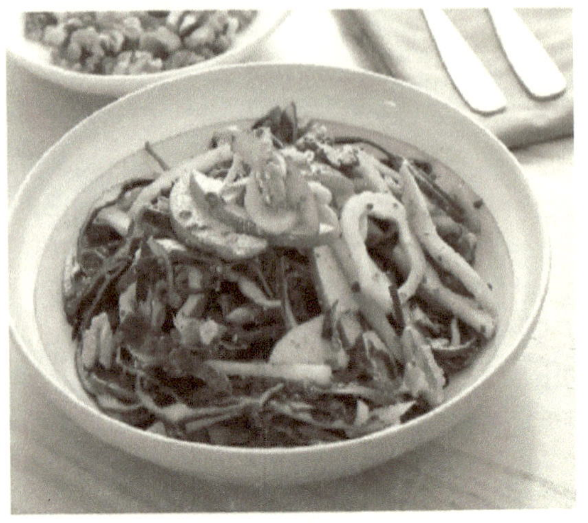

Serves: 4; Prep time: 10 minutes; Cooking time: 0 minutes; Total time: 10 minutes;

Nutritional values per serving:

Calories: 320 Cal; Fat: 28 g; Carbs: 15 g; Protein: 4 g; Fiber: 5 g;

Ingredients:

For the Dressing:

- 2 teaspoon minced ginger
- ¼ teaspoon ground black pepper
- 1/8 teaspoon red chili powder
- ¼ teaspoon salt
- 4 green cardamom pods, seeds ground

- 2 teaspoon erythritol sweetener
- 2 teaspoon Dijon mustard
- 6 tablespoons olive oil
- 2 tablespoon apple cider vinegar
- ½ of a lemon, juiced, zested

For the Salad:

- ½ cup ground almonds
- 1 medium organic mango, peeled, pitted, sliced
- 14 ounces shredded organic red cabbage

Instructions:

1. Prepare the dressing and for this, place all its ingredients in a small bowl and whisk until well combined.
2. Assemble the salad and for this, squeeze out moisture from sauerkraut as much as possible, then add it into a salad bowl, top with mango slices and sprinkle with almonds on top.
3. Drizzle prepared salad dressing over salad, toss until well mixed and serve.

Roasted Veggie Salad

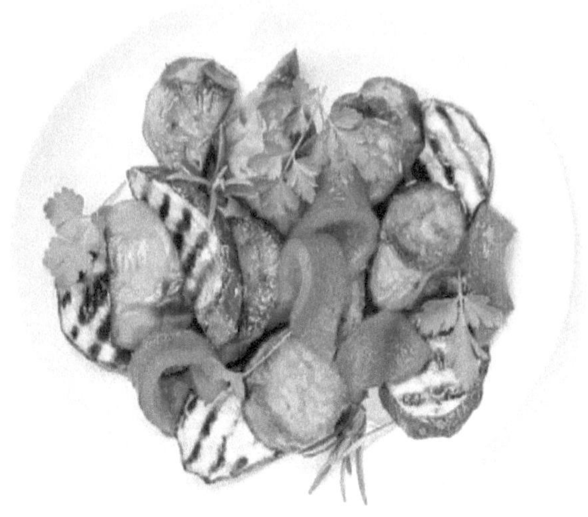

Serves: 4; Prep time: 10 minutes; Cooking time: 25 minutes; Total time: 35 minutes;

Nutritional values per serving:

Calories: 362 Cal; Fat: 14 g; Carbs: 55 g; Protein: 3.6 g; Fiber: 6.1 g;

Ingredients:

- 14 ounces organic potatoes, peeled
- 14 ounces organic sweet potatoes, peeled
- 14 ounces organic zucchini, peeled
- 4 tablespoons coconut oil, melted

  For the Salad Dressing:

- ½ cup apple cider vinegar

- 4 tablespoons date syrup

Instructions:

1. Switch on the oven, then set it to 350 degrees F, and let it preheat.
2. Meanwhile, cut potato, sweet potato, and zucchini into 1-inch pieces and add them in a baking sheet.
3. Drizzle oil over vegetables, then toss until well coated, spread the vegetables evenly in the baking sheet, and bake 25 minutes, flipping halfway through.
4. Meanwhile, prepare the salad dressing, and for this, whisk together vinegar and date syrup until combined.
5. When done, transfer roasted vegetables to a large salad bowl, drizzle with prepared dressing and toss until well coated.
6. Serve straight away.

Soups

Chicken and Chickpea Soup

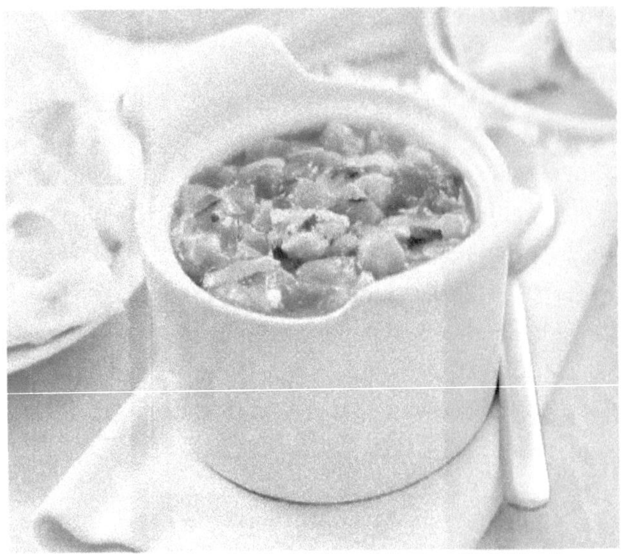

Serves: 4; Prep time: 10 minutes; Cooking time: 8 hours; Total time: 8 hours and 10 minutes;

Nutritional values per serving:

Calories: 446 Cal; Fat: 15 g; Carbs: 43 g; Protein: 34 g; Fiber: 12 g;

Ingredients:

- 1 cups dried chickpeas, soaked
- 1 ½ pounds antibiotic-free, pasteurized chicken thighs, skinless,

bone-in

- 12 ounces diced organic tomatoes, fire-roasted
- 10 ounces organic artichoke hearts, quartered
- 1 medium organic white onion , peeled, chopped
- 2 tablespoons halved organic olives, pitted
- 1 ½ teaspoons minced garlic
- ½ teaspoon salt
- ¼ teaspoon ground black pepper
- 3 teaspoons paprika
- 3 teaspoons ground cumin
- ¼ teaspoon cayenne pepper
- 1 bay leaf
- 1 ½ tablespoon tomato paste
- 3 cups of water
- 2 tablespoons chopped fresh cilantro

Instructions:

1. Drain chickpeas, place them in a 6-quarts slow cooker, then add tomatoes along with their juice, and rest of the ingredients except for olives, artichokes, cilantro, and salt and stir until well mixed.
2. Switch on the slow cooker, shut it with lid, and cook for 4 hours at high heat setting or 8 hours at low heat setting until thoroughly cooked.
3. When done, transfer chicken to a cutting board, let it cool for 5 minutes, and then shred with two forks.
4. Remove bay leaf from the soup, return chicken into the soup, add olives and artichokes and stir until mixed.
5. Garnish soup with cilantro and serve.

Chicken Zoodle Pho

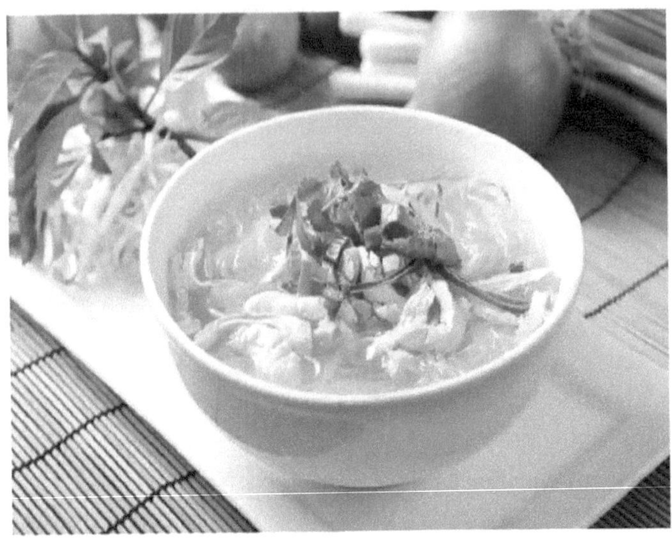

Serves: 4; Prep time: 10 minutes; Cooking time: 15 minutes; Total time: 25 minutes;

Nutritional values per serving:

Calories: 344.8 Cal; Fat: 11.5 g; Carbs: 19 g; Protein: 41.4 g; Fiber: 3.7 g;

Ingredients:

- 1 pound pasteurized chicken breast, cubed
- 1 cup of shredded organic carrot
- 2 cup organic zucchini noodles
- 2 cups sliced organic shitake mushrooms
- 2 teaspoons grated ginger

- ⅓ cup organic green onion, chopped
- 1 teaspoon minced organic garlic
- 1 tablespoon fish sauce
- 2 tablespoons lime juice
- 1 tablespoon coconut oil
- ½ cups coconut milk, unsweetened
- 4 cups of chicken bone broth
- ¼ cup chopped organic cilantro

Instructions:

1. Take a large pot, place it over medium heat, add oil and when it melts, add onion, carrot, ginger, carrot, and garlic and cook for 3 minutes until vegetable begins to soften.
2. Then add fish sauce, pour in milk and broth, stir well and bring the mixture to boil.
3. Switch heat to medium-low level, add chicken and simmer for 10 minutes until the chicken has thoroughly cooked.
4. Remove pot from heat, add lime juice and cilantro into the soup and stir until mixed.
5. Evenly divide zucchini noodles between four bowls, ladle soup over noodles and serve.

Emerald City Soup

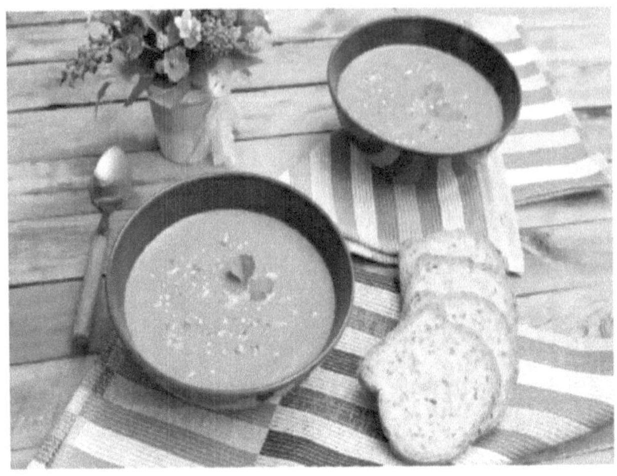

Serves: 4; Prep time: 10 minutes; Cooking time: 0 minutes; Total time: 10 minutes;

Nutritional values per serving:

Calories: 169.5 Cal; Fat: 7.7 g; Carbs: 20.8 g; Protein: 4.2 g; Fiber: 8.5 g;

Ingredients:

- 1 large organic avocado, peeled, pitted, diced
- 1 pound of fresh organic baby spinach
- 1 large bunch of organic cilantro, including stems
- 1 large organic cucumber
- 1 ½ cups chopped watermelon
- 2/3 cup coconut aminos
- 2 organic lemons, juiced

- 2/3 cup lime juice

Instructions:

1. Place all the ingredients in a food processor or blender and pulse for 2 to 3 minutes until smooth, scraping the sides.
2. Divide soup evenly between four bowls and serve.

Butternut Squash Soup

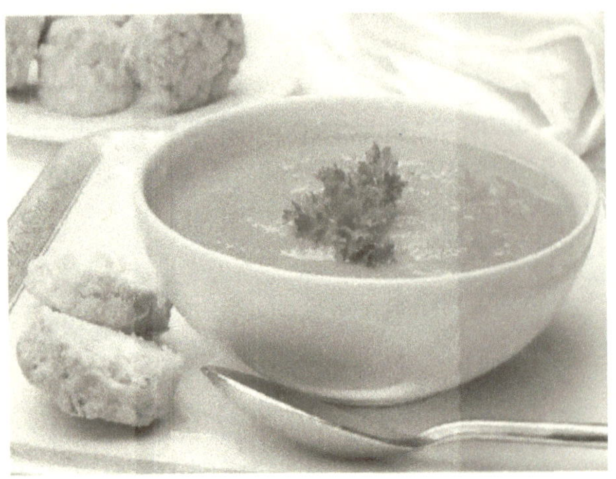

Serves: 4; Prep time: 10 minutes; Cooking time: 26 minutes; Total time: 36 minutes;

Nutritional values per serving:

Calories: 220 Cal; Fat: 7 g; Carbs: 34 g; Protein: 8.4 g; Fiber: 7.6 g;

Ingredients:

- 5 cups chopped organic butternut squash
- 1/2 teaspoon ginger powder
- 1 tablespoon minced organic garlic
- 1/2 teaspoon ground black pepper
- 1 teaspoon salt
- 1 teaspoon turmeric powder
- 1 tablespoon curry powder

- 1/2 tablespoon olive oil
- 2 cups of chicken bone broth
- 1/2 cup coconut milk, unsweetened
- Chopped organic parsley for topping

Instructions:

1. Take a large pot, place it over medium heat, add butternut squash, then pour in enough water to cover squash pieces by 1-inch and cook for 15 minutes until tender.
2. Drain the butternut squash and set aside until required.
3. Return pot over medium heat, add oil and when hot, add garlic and cook for 1 minute until fragrant.
4. Then add roasted butternut squash along with remaining ingredients, stir well and simmer for 10 minutes until thoroughly cooked.
5. Remove pot from heat, puree the soup by using an immersion blender until smooth and creamy and taste to adjust seasoning.
6. Ladle soup into four bowls, top with chopped parsley and serve.

Resources Page

Chapter 1

https://www.medicalnewstoday.com/articles/326117.php

https://www.medicalnewstoday.com/articles/326102.php

https://www.health.harvard.edu/blog/leaky-gut-what-is-it-and-what-does-it-mean-for-you-2017092212451

https://www.webmd.com/digestive-disorders/features/leaky-gut-syndrome

https://www.health.harvard.edu/diseases-and-conditions/the-gut-brain-connection

Chapter 2

https://www.webmd.com/digestive-disorders/what-your-gut-bacteria-say-your-health

https://www.mayoclinic.org/diseases-conditions/celiac-disease/symptoms-causes/syc-20352220

https://www.webmd.com/digestive-disorders/celiac-disease/celiac-disease

https://www.medicalnewstoday.com/articles/151620.php

https://chopra.com/articles/13-health-conditions-linked-to-the-gut-microbiome

https://www.thehealthy.com/digestive-health/disease-conditions-gut-bacteria/

Chapter 3

https://www.google.com/amp/s/www.hopkinsmedicine.org/health/wellness-and-prevention/the-brain-gut-connection%3famp=true

Chapter 4

https://thehealthychef.com/blogs/wellbeing/how-to-heal-your-gut-naturally

https://www.google.com/amp/s/www.psychologytoday.com/us/blog/click-here-happiness/201906/heal-the-gut-17-gut-healing-strategies-start-today%3famp

https://www.pcrm.org/health-topics/gut-bacteria

https://paleoleap.com/how-exercise-helps-with-gut-healing/

Chapter 5

https://www.medicalnewstoday.com/articles/326256.php

https://www.benenden.co.uk/be-healthy/nutrition/gut-food-15-foods-for-good-gut-health/

Chapter 6

https://www.thehealthy.com/food/eating-out-healthy/

https://www.verywellmind.com/what-is-a-mindset-2795025

www.ingramcontent.com/pod-product-compliance
Lightning Source LLC
Chambersburg PA
CBHW030312160726
47992CB00005B/1973